Praise for *Courage*

"Rachel has done a re
It takes courage to acco.............. ....p
into your courage today and go for your big goal that scares and
excites you. You'll be glad you did."

~ **Bob Proctor,** Teacher in *The Secret*,
Best Selling Author of *You Were Born Rich*

"I have said it before and I will say it again... Rachel Bazzy has
written one of the best books I have ever read. I am looking
forward to her sharing it with the world. She has a gift!"

~ **Peggy McColl**, *New York Times* Best Selling Author

"Rachel Bazzy and her story is one of loss, courage and true
personal transformation. She is now bringing the message of
courage to the world, seen through not only her own eyes, but also
through the eyes of other heroes. Get empowered, get courageous
and experience Real Magic by getting this book. Today!" "

~ **Anders Hansen,** Illusionist and
Transformational Speaker

"Fearlessly facing life. That is how I describe Rachel. If you want
to know what real courage is – the courage to LOVE deeply,
the courage to hold to your faith in your way, the courage to
face tragedy and HELP OTHERS in the process. If there is a
woman who has mastered the ART of being COURAGEOUS in
LIVING – it's Rachel. This book will unpack her heart and soul
in a MAP that gets you to COURAGEOUS LIVING AS WELL."

~ **Michael J Savage,** Master Coach & Facilitator
Robbins Research International,
an Anthony Robbins Company

"Courage is overcoming fear. It's a willingness to face agony, danger, uncertainty or intimidation and to take steps forward. For some it's getting out of bed in the morning or speaking with another, and for others, it's climbing a mountain or making the seeming impossible possible.

Rachel Bazzy has defined Courage and its many profiles with an understanding heart and amazing insight. This collection of stories presents real people who summoned their Courage to make it through incredible situations.

I have enormous respect for this woman, friend, and teacher who has endured tough circumstances. Rachel has written this book to help others understand courage, love, and faith as she has come to know them."

~ **Courtney Campbell,** Results Strategist,
Platinum Vision Inc.

"This book inspired me to courageously look within the deepest darkest depths of my soul in order to heal from the inside out."

~ **Wendy Ditta,** International Best Selling Author

"This book will show you how following your heart will lead you into new places. You will get a new perspective, and I always find that interesting and refreshing. If your fears are holding you back, this book is for you! If you suffer from anxiety, this book is for you! If you want to take control of your life, this book is for you!"

~ **Dr. Jussi Eerikäinen,** Cardiologist, Best Selling Author

"Rachel is one of the most courageous people I know. She has taken heartache after heartbreak and each time has chosen to rise. Deciding to rise, despite the fact that we've been beaten, knocked down, broken, and afraid... Choosing to pick ourselves up one moment at a time... We look around to discover one day

the clouds have lifted, the sun shines on our face, our feet have left the ground and we've learned how to fly. No matter where you stand today, **Courage** will give you the inspiration you need to get up until you can spread your wings and soar."

~ **Colleen Aynn,** International Bestselling Author of the *Feeling Friends* and Professional Speaker, Coach

"Great, just great! Rachel Bazzy's authenticity combined with her passionate writing style masterfully capture the reader and take them on a journey of self-discovery and awareness of the courage potential within all of us."

~ **Mick Petersen,** International Best Selling Author of *Stella and the Timekeepers*

"Have the courage to pick up a copy of this book for yourself, and buy one for a friend. This book has so many incredible examples of courage and the author, Rachel Bazzy is the epitome of courage herself. Rachel brings you on a journey to realize you have strength and the courage for whatever situation life deals you."

~ **Judy O'Beirn,** Creator of International Best Selling *Unwavering Strength* book series

"It was my honor to be interviewed by Rachel for her book on courage. I believe in working with people who are "walking the walk" and that is 100% of who Rachel is. Her perspectives are not untested theories or "feel good" analogies. She has walked through the fire and come out the other side with the beautiful scars that allow her to connect with people in a place of genuine compassion and understanding. I am blessed to know Rachel and filled with gratitude to be on this journey with her."

~ **Willard Barth**, Willard Barth Enterprises Licensed Master NAP Trainer & NLP Practitioner, Author, Business Consultant and Transformation Expert

"In the hero's journey, we learn that the journey is not finished as the hero must return to the original world and share what he or she has experienced. Thank you, Rachel, for bringing to us these beautiful examples of the 'return' and serving to build a strong belief in our individual courage and a trust in our intuition, allowing each one of us to push forward to the life we love living!"

  ~ **Kevin D. Smith,** Life Mastery Consultant
     International Best Selling Co-Author
     Chief Operating Officer of Andrew Mellen, Inc

"There are moments in life when we all could use some nuggets of inspiration to keep our faith in what's possible ignited progressively. May the excellent examples of COURAGE in this book of uplifting stories be an inspiring contribution to your growth."

  ~ **Callie K LeVina**

"The commitment of Rachel Bazzy to her readers is authentic and heartfelt. Her passion for lifting another's spirit through example is evident in this well-written collection of stories and lessons of courage. This has shifted my outlook on many of my daily stresses in a way that makes me feel like I can tackle and accomplish so much more."

  ~ **Brian Proctor,** VP of Business Development,
     Proctor Gallagher Institute
     Co-Author of *Darn Easy*

Permission should be addressed in writing to Rachel Bazzy at rachel@rachelbazzy.com

Editor: Sigrid Mcdonald
Book Magic, http://bookmagic.ca

Cover Design & Layout: Anne Karklins
anne@hasmarkpublishing.com

ISBN 13: 978-1-989756-24-9
ISBN 10: 1989756247

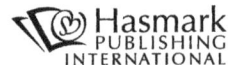

RACHEL BAZZY

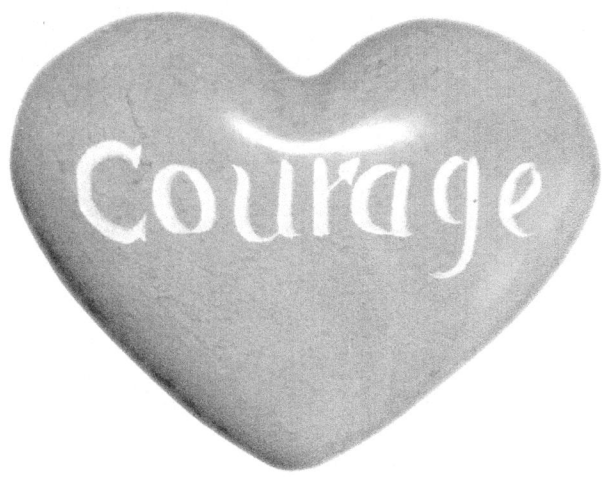

Master this,
and anything is possible.

FOREWORD BY PEGGY McCOLL
NEW YORK TIMES BEST SELLING AUTHOR

This book is dedicated to my husband, Chris,
who is my soulmate, my everything.
I also include our children in this dedication:
our daughter, Leah, and her husband, Nick, who is like a son;
our four grandchildren, Olivia, Isaak, Eden, and Ezra;
and our youngest son, Zach, and his girlfriend, Danielle.
I love all of you so much.

ACKNOWLEDGEMENTS

This book's idea was literally delivered to me through Spirit while I was taking a shower one morning! In the words of Alfred Adler, Austrian psychologist, "*I am grateful for the idea that has used me*". I acknowledge that Spirit, which is within all of us, that makes us One. I recognize my own courage which has developed in many areas of my life over the past two decades as I have studied and applied my knowledge of personal growth to my own life. I am grateful for my journey as a continuous seeker of enlightenment.

Along the way on this expedition called Personal Growth, I have had various teachers, instructors, and mentors who have guided me on my pathway. I am forever grateful for all of those who have served as mile-markers, road maps, GPS for the detours of Life, and encouraging counsel. I am grateful for people such as Michael Savage, Willard Barth, Rock Thomas, Sherry Sandford, and my amazing friend, Dr. Jussi Eerikäinen. I have learned incredible lessons along my journey from masters like Tony Robbins and Bob Proctor, and the legacy works and wisdom of Earl Nightingale, Dr. Joseph Murphy, Napoleon Hill, Thomas Troward, James Allen, and Neville Goddard, to name a few.

I am incredibly grateful for my mentor, Peggy McColl, who has taught me how to navigate the literary world, and continues to teach, encourage, and advise me. Thank you, Peggy, for believing in me. I treasure our destiny together.

I am surrounded with a circle of elite friends, collaborators, peers, and affiliates, all of whom hold me and each other in accountability. There are so many whom I cherish and am grateful for, however, I would be remiss if I did not mention my reading partner, Kevin Smith, dear friend and sounding board, Wendy Ditta, and my accountability partner, Al Proctor. I love you guys to the moon!

My passion for writing and teaching is thankfully backed by a team of technical supporters: to my publisher and friend, Judy O'Beirn at Hasmark Publishing, I thank you so much! And for Judy's fabulous team: Jenn Gibson, you are a jewel; Michelle Mifsud, you are priceless. My beautiful book cover design was created by Anne Karklins, who really captured my vision for the cover, and to my editor, Sigrid MacDonald, I say thank you so very much; I truly enjoyed working with you.

I hold a special appreciation for our son Zach Bazzy for his design and building my webpage. I especially am grateful for his understanding that when Mom lacks technical jargon, he gets it intuitively. And for my attorney, beautiful Banafsheh Akhlaghi, I hold you in high esteem; thank you for having my back.

I am very appreciative of all of those who have shared their story of courage with me in this book. I am absolutely honored to be entrusted with the biography of your heart. You are a testimony to the spirit of mankind; not just in surviving but in thriving beyond the adversity in your lives. You are examples of hope and Light for all of those who will read this book, and I thank you from my soul.

I am so happy and grateful for my readers and the lives which are being creatively transformed through higher understanding and awareness. May you all be encouraged to seek and fulfill your dreams and true destinies.

Most importantly, I am grateful for Chris, my loving husband of over 40 years, who loves me, my silliness, still thinks I'm cute, and supports me in every endeavor. You complete me.

"Surround yourself with the dreamers and the doers,
the believers and the thinkers, but most of all,
surround yourself
with those who see greatness within you,
even when you don't see it yourself."

~ Edmund Lee, Author

In Memory

Of our son,
Eric Christopher Bazzy
March 16, 1980 – November 13, 2015

I see you in the rainbow,
I hear you in the wind;
The stars glitter like your mischievous eyes,
All untouchable, to my chagrin.

Your voice is in my head,
Your laughter a memory dear;
I love you and I miss you, son,
Yet, I know you are always near.

Come see me in my slumber,
Come hug me in my dreams;
Let me see your handsome face once more,
In the sunshine and moonbeams.

The ocean crashes at my feet,
The wind blows through my hair;
Whenever I see a rainbow, son,
I know that you are there.

~ Mom

Poem by Rachel Bazzy

TABLE OF CONTENTS

Foreword
by Peggy McColl

For many years, I have been blessed to train and mentor authors; providing them with the guidance to write their books, publish, self-publish, make their books best sellers and build their businesses doing work that is deeply meaningful. One of the blessings of working with authors is the way that their books bring so much value to the world. This book is no exception. Rachel Bazzy has created one of my absolute favorite books of all time. I absolutely LOVE this book.

Without a doubt, I believe this book will bring a tremendous amount of value to the world. Period. This is a book that you will read and reread, and, if you are smart, you'll buy copies for everyone you care about.

You see, courage is something that we can all use a little more of. There have been, are, and will be, times in our lives when we are faced with fear. It is during those times that we need to be able to be equipped to effectively manage the potentially destructive emotion (fear). I believe, with the creative and clever way Rachel constructed this book, you will not only be inspired but you will be well equipped to handle fear and turn it to courage.

When Rachel asked me about moments in my own life when I faced fear, several past experiences came to mind. "Do I have to choose just one?" I asked jokingly. In this book, Rachel is sharing one of my own "fear-to-courage" moments that was heart wrenching (I won't say what it was, as you have the book to refer to in the chapter called: "The Courage to Let Go"). Rachel also shares many courageous stories of others she interviewed and these stories will have you awestruck.

My recommendation is that you dedicate the time to really dive into the depths of this book … really study it. You will very likely relate to some of the stories and reminisce about the times when you had to go within to find your courage.

Courage is something that we all have. We may not recognize courage at the time that we need it, but it is there nonetheless. And, if you are looking for strategies to move from fear to courage, you'll also find them in this book.

Without hesitation, it is time for you to go to the opening chapter. Get started now. I would like to wrap up this foreword with one word of caution… you may become so captivated that you will find the time simply flies by. You may find that you read this book in one sitting; and come back to it later to catch more of the highlights.

Enjoy this courageous journey.

Peggy McColl
http://PeggyMcColl.com

Introduction

November 13, 2015

"Hello?"

I answered my cell phone that night from an unknown caller; it was a number I didn't recognize, but coming from a nearby, small town that I was quite familiar with. My senses were suddenly heightened.

"Mrs. Bazzy?"

My heart beat faster. I knew that tone of voice. I had heard it countless times back when we were raising our three teenagers. I had become accustomed to the late night voice of a local authority, calling to alert us of some misdemeanor or infraction, a traffic incident or prank-gone-askew, and always needing one of us to either come post bail or take the guilty kid home to discipline with our own restrictions and consequences. As my mind quickly recalled all the scenarios of the past, I also knew in real time, that our "kids" were no longer kids. They were in their 30's, two of them married, and all of them happy and responsible adults.

"Yes?", I responded cautiously.

The man's voice was calibrated as he asked if we had a son named Eric Bazzy. I affirmed. I was keenly aware that Eric was on a road trip on his motorcycle, heading towards the hill country for a friend's wedding the next day. I didn't like where this conversation was leading. A whirring of thoughts ran through my mind, as the man identified himself as the chaplain of the little town's hospital. It was the same little town, and the same little hospital, that Eric was taken to years ago, when he had made a suicide attempt. This night, now sober, he was headed to the exact town farther north, where he had spent time in recovery after that incident. The irony was not lost on me. I drew in a deep breath and subconsciously held it, fortifying myself.

The chaplain hem-hawed around, mincing his words, delicately attempting to ask if we could come to the hospital. My intuition was in overdrive. I felt sorry for this poor, gentle soul, who was stumbling through his attempt at tactfulness. I knew what he was trying not to say. By now, my ears were ringing. My heart was pounding in my throat. My patience and usual phone courtesy suddenly snapped; I interrupted the cryptic rambling, and exhaled my demand:

"Is he dead?"

"Well, ma'am, uh…", he stammered on.

"*Just tell me. I can take it. Just spit it out! IS. HE. DEAD?*"

There was a coarse silence before the pronouncement confirmed every parent's worst nightmare. My heart lurched, stomach churned. I asked "how", but I already knew. Our family loved motorcycles and we had shared the enthusiasm and love of riding for years. The chaplain began to explain there was an accident, and where it happened, but by then my mind was too traumatized to process the details.

What seemed like a quickening few seconds of conversation now became a time stop. I handed the phone to my husband and stumbled in slow motion to the bathroom. Tears of denial mixed with the bile of anger as I spat into the toilet. I violently pounded the seat, screaming the words, "NO, NO, NO!", over and over again. I was enraged. I felt cheated. I refused to accept .it. It was unbelievable, unacceptable. I was numb.

~

December 13, 2017

Years later, while working on the manuscript for this book, I reread the original introduction, which I had written much earlier, and I hated it. It felt contrived, ordinary. I now had a better vision for the message of this book, and I was pressing my timeline to complete the manuscript for my publisher. I realized I needed to scrap the first version of the introduction and began anew from a place in time where this subject began for me. No, I didn't decide to write a book because of that fateful night, however, the day Eric died, something in me was born. And I had been unconsciously gestating it for years. Courage.

Courage I hadn't recognized I possessed. Courage of an entirely different caliber. A spirit of courage that had to be summoned from a place outside of myself. Courage from my subconscious mind.

Look, our son's death was a terrible, traumatic event in the lives of our family, our friends, and ourselves. It was going to take some undefined amount of time to heal my heart's wound. There were many days when that wound was very tender, and I experienced melancholy, and cried easily. But as time went on, the space grew longer between those depressions of grieving and my recovering heart. I learned to recognize the triggers, the environment, and the seemingly common, everyday events and conversations that provoked a private meltdown. I developed the courage to let go of those entitlements, and heal myself. I chose to focus on my gratitude for everything in my life, and in the life of our son. I learned not to pick at the scab. I developed the courage along the way, and let it heal. I will never be over our son's death, but I am continually growing stronger, through this event of my life.

When rewriting this introduction, I realized that I was making myself vulnerable to the grief frequency, through my thoughts. The more I thought about that night, recalled the story so I could write about it, the more my body manifested the vibration of that event. I found that, once again, my heart was pounding, and I felt cold and clammy. I could feel my spirit sinking, getting sucked into the vortex of loss and sadness. I was circling the drain again. That paradigm of grief, sadness, and loss was pulling at me, like an undercurrent that would suck me in deeper and deeper.

Nearly in tears, I stopped writing. I forced myself to calm down. I changed my physicality; walked around, ate something, talked to my husband, got out some essential oils, listened to my meditation audio. That grief paradigm fought back a little, but I quickly kicked its ass. I *chose* to take the actions necessary to pull myself back up to a higher frequency.

I made a conscious decision to change my vibration.

I have a burning desire to teach you how to do the same thing. I am here to help you. My intent in this book is to teach you to recognize the courage that lies within yourself, develop courage in every aspect of your life, and master any and all situations in your life. You must develop courage, if you want to succeed in Life. I am here to help you.

This book offers you a collection of stories, examples, and quotes to support your personal growth. The goal is to aid you in discovering your strengths, and guide you away from the fear that keeps you from developing this essential human trait. I am here to mentor you along your journey of self-discovery, awakening, and development of your courage and your mind.

I encourage you to not only read, but also study this book. Tell a friend about this book. We are all here to bring the light of our Creator into fuller expression, to bring love and hope, and lift one another up. My intention for you is that you will connect with the spirit in which this book has been written. I have written it with love for you, because I know the potential you have, that we all have, to expand in knowledge, understanding, and personal growth.

I honor the place in you that is the same in me.
I honor the place in you where the whole universe resides.
I honor the place in you of love, of light, of peace and truth.
I honor the place in you that is the same in me.
There is but One.

Namaste

ONE

Courage in a Box

Not often enough, our attention is brought to the story of a child who has been recognized for displaying incredible courage in the face of adversity. I believe we should focus more on these positive, inspiring examples of courage, and pay less attention to the negative news and drama that is served up on daily media. Focusing on the positive brings more positive into our lives and the lives of others.

One example of courage is in persevering in the face of adversity. Tremendous courage is seen in those children who face disease, medical diagnosis, and special needs. These young warriors accept each day as a gift as they bravely strive to conquer their daily challenges. Their siblings and caretakers often fall into the category of unsung heroes, as the family goes through a long-lasting battle against the odds. Courage in all is strengthened even more by the endurance they exhibit, and through the love and support of others around them.

There is immeasurable courage in the kids who have displayed heroic efforts to save the life of another person, and uncommon courage in those who selflessly put their own life at risk to save someone else's life. We see time and again the hero whose only thought was, "I love my dad (or mom or friend); I didn't want him to die". It doesn't get much more basic than love, doing the right thing, and following your heart.

There are young athletes who persevere through hardship or disadvantage. We draw inspiration from the accounts of their sporting achievements, despite the physical or mental challenges, regardless of poverty, undeterred by great loss or disaster.

Gratefully, today there are organizations and programs that recognize and promote the courageous hearts of children, but not everyone's story gets shared or acknowledged. I am going to share the story of a very special little boy, as a gift to you, because his story has been a gift to me.

> *"Courage is about doing what you're afraid to do.*
> *There can be no courage unless you are scared.*
> *Have the courage to act instead of react."*

~ Eddie Rickenbacker, WWI American Flying Ace

Imagine that your parents are refugees from Finland, displaced by an invasion from the Soviet Union, and now exist in the unfamiliarity of a cramped, poor ghetto. In these very meager conditions, the supplies, food and medicine are scarce. Overcrowded with women and children, the men are tired and frustrated, scrounging daily for meager jobs to support their families. Imagine that your older siblings and you are born into this abject poverty, into this adversity, and are raised with hatred: an unholy hatred for the enemy who uprooted everyone's lives. In this environment of bitterness, anxiety, lack, and longing, your family life also includes a mother with mental illness, and verbal and physical abuse sparked by episodes of unbalance, frustrations, and exaggerated delusions. Thus, the life of little Jussi began.

Underweight and small for his age, Jussi's big blue eyes were accentuated by his small frame. Little Jussi was quiet and introverted, and at a young age, through his perception, he quickly learned how to "lay low", so as not to stir up anything with his mother when she was having 'an episode'. The only area he seemed unable to control was his night terrors. As he cried out in his nightmares, his mother would express her own fears through anger and violence by beating him with a belt to awaken him. At other times, she kept his toys from him as discipline, deeming his minor, childish mistakes as mortal, grave sins, worthy of severe punishment.

Jussi grew, quietly observing everything around him. Curiously thinking and calculating, he was always looking for answers. As his consciousness grew, he began picking up on the tremulous vibration of his parents as they hashed over the difficult decisions that would affect their lives. He listened intently as his parents fantasized out loud about escaping to a better life. Jussi stretched his imagination and tried to visualize what a better life would look like, too.

Imagine then, that one day, when Jussi's father set out to find that better life and boarded a ship for unknown lands. Father and son said their tearful goodbyes, and he was gone. Jussi was filled with fear; the fear of being left with his mother, who had been diagnosed with a mental disorder. With no voice of reason in the house, no protector, and the exaggerated drama in his mother's head, his life seemed out of his control. He clung to the memories of his father reading *Robinson Crusoe* to him, explaining science, and quoting Albert Einstein. To Jussi, his father was his hero, an adventurer and role model, despite his occasional drinking binges.

Eventually, Jussi's father found work in Colombia, South America, with a British gold mining company. With the promise of a good salary and safe housing, he worked diligently for months and months, saving his salary until he had enough to purchase the one-way tickets on an ocean liner that would reunite him with his young family.

The day came when, with wide-eyes and trepidation, Jussi recalls having boarded the enormous ocean liner with his weepy mother. Their modest cabin was more luxurious than anything he had ever seen in his short life, yet it felt like a prison to him. He was boxed in. Feeling fearful to leave the only home he'd ever known, he was even more frightened to be in this small space with his deranged mother. He was sequestered in the cabin, staying with his mother and her neurosis. She bemoaned and wept the entire trip. Jussi felt helpless, with no refuge, and no protection from her volatile behavior or outbursts.

Banging and groaning noises resounded from the bowels of the ship. On a rare occasion, Jussi found himself on an upper deck. Looking outwards, he felt the incredible isolation of the vessel being in the middle of a huge, endless sea. As he gazed across the immense waters, his eyes searched beyond the horizon; it was limitless. He studied the sky; it was infinite. He closed his eyes and dreamed he was flying. He felt free.

The long, trans-Atlantic journey finally deposited them in a strange land of heat and humidity, strange foods, even stranger clothing, and dark-skinned people who spoke a foreign language that none of them could understand.

Imagine being this young boy now living in the jungles of Colombia. It was all so completely different from his previous world. He was free from the poverty of the ghetto. He had room to breathe. New sounds coaxed his ears, new smells tantalized his nostrils, and so much to explore and learn: a totally new environment!

And, not so new. The same vibration of anxiety and fear emitted from Jussi's parents, as they whispered their worries to one another after lights out. Jussi could grasp snatches of hushed conversation, and the fear of another psychotic episode from his mother kept him awake at night. He would hear the words 'guerrillas' and 'Soviet Union' which caught his attention. Names like Fidel Castro, Jorge Gaitan, and Bogotá hung in the thick, sultry air. Then suddenly without warning, his family was secretly whisked away to a new city, relocated *again!* Jussi believed that and he and his parents were in grave danger because the communists that his parents hated so passionately were disrupting the mining operations in the jungles.

Life was better in the urban city of Bogotá, until Jussi contracted a severe bacterial infection in his skull. The Mastoiditis then infected his kidneys. He was a very sick little boy. Bedridden for 14 months, he endured injections three times a day, and the occasional nursing from his distracted mother. He did his school studies from his mattress. Jussi idolized Albert Einstein and wanted to grow up to be a nuclear physicist just like him. He persevered in his schooling and in his physical rehabilitation.

Back in the 1940s, living in a destabilizing region of Colombia, young Jussi was in charge of his own rehab. He taught himself to crawl first, then, as his strength returned, he learned to walk all over again. When he was able, he returned to attend a private, Catholic school in the city of Bogotá, where his family had relocated. Schoolboy Jussi, still skinny and now wearing over-sized eyeglasses, attended his classes with a new zest for learning. He had a genius level of understanding in math and science and wanted to understand how the world worked. He was bullied by the local children who did not share his enthusiasm; his intellect was misunderstood.

And yet, he learned to adapt and enjoy this new urban life, despite the political turbulence in the adult world. Jussi loved the parks, the open markets, and especially the wonderful museums. Then as quickly, it seemed, as he had adapted to his new environment, the city was under assault by the leftist insurgents who filtered down from the Colombian jungles and mountains.

By the late 1940s, the communists' efforts in Bogotá were being led by Jorge Eliecer Gaitan, a charismatic, political revolutionary. A young, Cuban socialist named Fidel Castro was on his was way to Colombia, to organize events against the Pan-American Student's Conference, which were taking place there in April, 1948. With communist leanings and affiliations, based on historic accounts, Castro met with Gaitan once, before being arrested and interrogated for impudently distributing leaflets protesting various, political issues. The atmosphere was charged like an electrical storm, made up of politics, terror, and chaos.

The climate of the city of Bogotá was very unstable. On April 9, 1948, Jorge Eliecer Gaitan was assassinated on the very day he was scheduled to meet again with Fidel Castro. His murder set off *massive riots* and escalating violence that destroyed much of downtown Bogotá. Castro joined the fighting in the streets. The place resembled a bombed target, as government buildings were set on fire and vehicles burned; *thousands* of people were killed in confrontation. This day, known in history known as "*El Bogatazo*" (meaning, The Violent Augmentation), sparked a 50 year-long period of Colombian civil war. The historical violence, known as "*La Violencia*" (The Violence) which followed, spread rapidly across the entire country, with over 300,000 documented deaths, and nearly eight million Colombians displaced within their own borders.

Prior to the assassination, Jussi was informed that his father had been approached by the Americans, who enlisted him in helping defeat the leftist presidential candidate, Jorge Eliecer Gaitan. Fueled by his long-held anger for this enemy, the communists, he had agreed. Years of unsettled, brewing political turmoil was now at a boiling point in the city, and it burned in the soul of Jussi's father and other Conservative supporters. He secretly joined the ranks of the conspirators.

After the assassination, eventually Jussi's father got wind of the danger he and his family were in. He assigned Jussi and his mother to pack suitcases for their escape. Once more, they were going to relocate. Jussi felt his father's hatred towards the communists for forcing them to flee once again; the tension was palatable. Jussi perceived that his mother was going into another breakdown, as the two of them threw articles of clothing into bags. Outside the home, Jussi heard a truck approach. He bristled at the sounds of loud shouting, and a sense of warning instinctively gnawed in his gut.

Suddenly, in retaliation for their suspected involvement in their leader's death, an angry cartel of commando guerrillas burst into their home and brutally *kidnapped* Jussi and his parents. They blindfolded all three of the family members, and dragged them from their home. They were hastily driven over bumpy roads and rutted trails, deep into the mountains beyond civilization. Jussi's mother hunched down next to him, silently weeping, while his own heart pounded in his throat. His ominous dread was beyond words. Fear shook him to his core, fracturing his sense of being, numbing his young mind.

Finally, the vehicle came to a rough stop. The engine ticked in a heated protest as the rain fell in a drenching downpour. Jussi and his parents were roughly shoved out of the vehicle and made to stand in the deluge. Abruptly their hoods were removed. Jussi squinted against the sudden, watery light, his breathing erratic. He felt very small. Trapped in this narrow clearing by his father's nemesis, he could barely register their hardened faces and menacing posture. Somewhere deep inside, though, he could feel their hatred. He held his breath, attempting to stop the tremors in his small frame.

The Comandante shouted the order, "*MATALOS!* Kill them!" In horror and utter disbelief, Jussi watched as his parents were violently pushed down on their knees into the mud. Before his mind could register the sounds of the rifles' chambering, he was involuntarily flinching from the sudden explosion of gunfire. Jussi's parents were executed right in front of him, their blood mingling with the mud and the rain, pooling around his feet. With the crack of gunshot still ringing in his ears, he went into shock. His world turned surreal. No ten-year-old kid should have to see this. As he collapsed to his knees, a man from behind grabbed him and jerked him back up. Jussi stood there, alone. Orphaned and terrified, his hot tears intermixed with the rain and the blood of his parents. His life had been unexplainably spared, but all he wanted to do was die.

Dragged to his feet, Jussi was forced to march through the mountain jungles, in the pouring rain for hours and hours. His mind reeled. His head was spinning, his breathing labored. His thin little body shivered uncontrollably. Unconsciously, he put one foot in front of the other as he stumbled along the darkening path, surrounded by these merciless executioners. When they finally reached a crude base camp, Jussi was cast into a small cage like an animal.

For well over a week, Jussi sat in his prison, numb with grief. Traumatized, he slumped over, reliving the barbarity of his parents' deaths, continuously sobbing as the scene played over and over in his mind, until there were no more tears. The nights were black, filled with unknown foes and noises. The days were tedious, filled with rainfall, shouting, and uncertainty. One of the cooks, a middle-aged woman with long, dark hair, took pity on the young boy. She delivered his food with compassion in her eyes. On the tenth evening, when she brought his meal, she quietly breathed a message to Jussi; "I can help you escape if you promise to follow my directions exactly as I tell you". The violence and bloodshed had left Jussi leery and suspicious. The kind woman must have sensed his hesitation. She coaxed him, "Trust in me. I will help you". Then she disappeared into the darkness.

Jussi waited anxiously for the next few days. Nothing happened. He began to think perhaps he had imagined the suggested escape. He searched his mind for clarity. Meanwhile, the kindhearted woman used her charms on one of the guerrillas who was in love with her. She leveraged his desires and convinced him to collaborate with her in her tactics to help Jussi escape. The guerrilla member shared the camp schedule with her, and the knowledge of their comings and goings. One evening at twilight, she brought the meal to Jussi as usual, sat it on the ground, and paused. She and Jussi locked eyes. "It is time to make your escape", she whispered matter-of-factly, as she took his hand and led him away quickly. She gave him instructions as they walked, but his mind was racing.

"Tell me again!" Jussi begged, but she shook her head no.

"But, I don't understand…"

They stopped at the edge of the camp, where she assured him, "Don't worry, you'll understand my instructions when you need to". Jussi stood gazing at this angel of mercy, memorizing her kind face, wondering where she came from... Suddenly, there was movement in the distance. Jussi froze, not sure what to do.

"RUN!" she hissed as she shoved him towards the dense forest. Gunfire rang out and bullets ricocheted off the trees around him. Malnourished and traumatized, he somehow found the courage and strength to run as fast as he could, knowing his life depended on it. The rounds whizzed past his head as he plunged forward down the barely visible path. As he ran, he glanced and saw the steep embankment she had warned him about. Without hesitating, he plummeted down the drop-off and into a dense jungle, so thick and dark he could barely see. Shadows became imagined foes, as he quietly fumbled his way in the underbrush until he found his refuge hidden within. *A wooden box!* Just as the cook had promised him, here was his salvation. He slipped inside the hiding place and tried to control his breathing. Cursed shouts and the booted footsteps of the guerilla force echoed off the trees and rocks. With every sound, Jussi would draw in his breath, shivering in fear that his hiding place had been discovered. He lay perfectly still, his mind racing. What would they do to him if they discovered him? He pictured the terrifying possibilities in his active imagination, as he tried to shrink himself into the dark corners of his trunk.

As the dark settled in for the night, and the angry sounds faded away, Jussi lay thinking. He wondered if he would survive this wretchedness. Having never really had much use for his Catholic school's religious liturgy, he now prayed in his own way. He pleaded with God to let him live. He was convinced that his destiny couldn't end this way! *Please, God, help me make it out alive*, he repeated, over and over.

Jussi's guardian angel showed up in the form of a small, green frog. The little fellow calmly jumped upon Jussi's arm and wouldn't leave his new friend. His peacefulness bewildered the ten-year-old boy. The frog didn't seem to feel any fear, so it must be something that Jussi was doing to himself, he figured. He discovered that the fear he felt was on the inside, that he had created the fear internally; it was not on the outside. The little, green frog had a calm energy that Jussi held onto, as he lay there thinking. Eventually, he developed three ideas that he would live by for the rest of his life:

(1) Everything is energy.

(2) No matter the situation, as long as he maintained a calmness of mind, he'd get through it.

(3) Everything was in his head, and he had the power to control situations with his thoughts.

Courage, in a box. Imagine that.

The moment Jussi decided to release his fear and activate his courage, a feeling of confidence swept over him. He knew that he would survive this ordeal. He finally felt safe. His confidence grew. Ten-year-old Jussi, wise beyond his years, had found inner peace.

While in his hideaway trunk struggling to come to terms with the tragedy of his parents' death and the loss of everything in his life, Jussi also felt the conflicting feeling of freedom from his mother's psychosis. Although later in his life he would suffer with PTSD (post-traumatic stress disorder) until he healed himself, Jussi's young mind now found refuge in a certain *knowing* that he would never be beaten awake with a belt again.

Long after dark had settled on the second day filled with rain, Jussi creaked open the lid of the trunk, peeked out, and then stood up gingerly. His body was stiff and sore from the damp hiding place, and he was hungry and dehydrated. His companion, the little, green frog, jumped casually to a nearby branch, and stared back at Jussi one last time. He seemed to say, "Go in peace".

Scampering through the wet shadows like a night creature, Jussi picked his way through the unfamiliar scenery until he came upon a small village. Weak and thirsty, the feeling of a total collapse overtook him. In the distance, a woman was motioning for him to come to her modest house. Jussi summoned what courage and strength he had left and stumbled towards the stranger's door. The gentle woman quickly drew him in with no explanation necessary. She fed him and gave him water to restore him, before hiding him away so he could rest. She arranged for a bus ride with her brother, to go back to the capitol city of Bogotá.

The bus drove along the long, bumpy road towards Bogotá with the possibility of encountering guerillas soldiers. With every lurch, every screeching brake tap, Jussi could feel the fear of being recaptured rise within himself. He would start worrying about being taken back to their camp and tortured or killed. Eventually, as Jussi realized his wondering thoughts took him to these dark places, he learned to redirect his mind, think of the frog, and of his three convictions, and the fear would pass.

The bus ride ended at the unsafe downtown depot. The now off-duty driver compassionately drove Jussi across town to a Catholic school, the only safe place Jussi could think of. Gratefully, he shook the driver's hand, then stepped out into the dusty street. Weakly, he mounted the steps, then curled up by the front door of the school and slept until the headmistress discovered him the next morning. She and the other staff members cried with compassion as Jussi described the horrible ordeal he had survived. They took him in, nurtured him, and later arranged for an introduction to a wonderful German family, who eventually adopted Jussi as their own.

Being with his new family felt like paradise to Jussi. Here he had the freedom to dream, the open-minded atmosphere to grow, and continue his music, sketching, and painting. Being in this family was a gift. He was safe. His new mama spoiled him with affection. He felt loved, secure, and accepted. And, he finally had a voice. He pushed the personal tragedy of his parents' deaths into the back of his mind. Only at night, when he lay awake thinking and feeling alone, would he explore those dark memories, feeling those emotions once again. For years, he silently cried himself to sleep.

Jussi became ill one day after joining his new family. He had a little retreat in the upper loft of their home, and tucked himself away up there, not feeling well. When Mama and Papa discovered he was not about his usual routine, they sought to find him. They climbed up and discovered him shivering in his loft. Papa descended to go get some water and a cool rag. Mama was a kind, gentle, loving woman, very wise, and very protective of Jussi. She climbed all the way up the ladder-like steps and into the loft, inquiring about the matter with her boy. She placed her hand on his hot forehead. Realizing he was running a high fever and seeing his misery, she was full of sympathy, cooing and cuddling him closely, drawing his head to rest on her bosom, as so many moms do. He could hear her heart beating. It was profound. He had never been cuddled or loved like this, never felt this protected. In fact, he had never heard another's heartbeat. He sat in his dearest mama's arms and sobbed and sobbed with gratitude for her love.

Jussi continued to flourish in his home environment, but his health and grades suffered. He was often sick; he suffered an aneurysm, had bouts of paralysis on the right side of his body, was bullied at school, and had no friends. He was haunted with questions about his survival, about the injustice that happened to his parents and himself, and their horrific deaths that he had witnessed. As he matured, he questioned his own destiny. Did all of that chaos he was raised with make him who he was? Did it prepare him for life, somehow? Could living without his parents somehow make him stronger?

About this time in his life, in some serendipitous way, he acquired a recording by Earl Nightingale titled *The Strangest Secret*. Jussi was intrigued by the message and listened to it repeatedly. The truths spoken began to make sense to him. He ran home from school every day, excited to listen to the message, again and again. Eventually, Jussi's life began to change. He decided to focus on his studies and gradually, his grades improved. His outlook improved; the bullying stopped, he made friends, and gained confidence in himself. That same sense of calmness filled him, much like the peace he felt years ago when he met the frog in the box. Answers were coming for the soulful questions that had haunted him for years. Albert Einstein's explanation about energy being everything began to help Jussi make sense of things. As his awareness of an ever-present, invisible energy grew, he felt connected to something bigger than himself, and he wanted to understand what it was. From tragedy to triumph, he went on to attend university, excelling in mathematics and eventually earning his doctorate in medicine (M.D.).

Dr. Jussi Eerikäinen has gone on to live an incredible life as an extra-ordinary mathematician and cardiologist. He turned his childhood goal of becoming a nuclear physicist, like Einstein, into a courageous passion for helping others. For more than 30 years, he practiced both traditional and alternative methods of healing while living in Venezuela. Through the study and research of energy, morphic fields, signature frequencies, and our human brain, Dr. Jussi and his creative thinking led him to treat patients all over the world with energy, frequency, and prevention. Once again, escaping communism, he now resides in the safety of Tenerife, Canary Islands with his dear, sweet wife, Ramonita. I cannot imagine a more generous, sweet, selfless couple than Jussi and Ramonita. It is a privilege to call them both my dear, beloved friends. I am deeply honored to share the story of Jussi's courage and persistence.

Dr. Jussi continues to study, teach, and design programs that are changing the lives of humanity all over the world. His latest book, *Transforming Vibes*, is an International Best Seller, which I highly recommend.

For more information on his incredible work, go to VibrantResults.com

TWO

THE COURAGE TO LIVE

My magnificent publisher and friend, Judy O'Beirn, is one of the most heroic, compassionate women I know. I am continually amazed by her courage, her faith, and her unwavering strength. And the best part is, she has deeper reservoirs of courage that she doesn't even realize are there! I see it in her, I hear it in her voice, and I read it in between the lines of her writings. She keeps me centered, in serene ways that she may not even be aware of.

"A hero is an ordinary individual who finds the strength to persevere and endure in spite of overwhelming obstacles"

~ Christopher Reeve

Judy and I were talking, one rainy day, about one of her books that includes her incredible story of the unprecedented courage she found to endure the loss of those she loved. I had read her book, *Unwavering Strength*, which is filled with exceptional stories, and I was deeply touched by her fortitude, her strength, and her commitment to help others. I mentioned to Judy that I wanted to include part of her story in my next book titled *Courage*, which I was currently writing. She just smiled, rolled her beautiful eyes towards the heavens and shrugged, when I referred to her own courageous journey.

"You know, I don't know. Haha, hahaha. I don't think I would have wanted to know what was coming, because I would have said, NO WAY. No way do I have the courage to go through *that*."

My response was, "That is why it is a good thing we don't know what is coming, or we would waste all of our time dreading it, instead of living our life". Judy smiled, and nodded her head in a knowing response.

I have certainly lived my own sentiment. I hadn't even considered the level of courage I was going to need when our oldest son, Eric, was suddenly killed on his motorcycle at the age of 32. I went into a tailspin. Our entire family dynamic was changed in a nanosecond, by a bump in the night. It seemed like I couldn't process it fast enough, and the pain was excruciating and cruel. I wanted to wake up from the nightmare and realize it was all just a bad dream.

There is NO preparation for any type of tragic news. Even being a bystander, or more importantly, a caregiver, for a loved one who is imprisoned in a diseased body, is no less preparatory for their death than those of us who have suffered a sudden loss. If ever there was grace, it is this from our Maker: the blissful ignorance of dates, times, and events, which physically rob us of those whom we treasure. It is better that we live our lives in the awareness of our love and gratitude for all those whom we cherish, and live each day to its fullest.

My husband and I have found a way to get through that tragic event, by focusing on our gratitude for all the good in our lives, and the gratefulness we have for being Eric's parents.

We choose to look outside of ourselves through contribution and service to other people in various ways. We have metered out our grieving; it's only a little over two years, at the time of this writing. Some days, some moments, just *suck*. Even as I write this, it reconnects me to that feeling of disbelief, longing, and sadness. We have both had to learn that the "trick" is not to stay stuck in that vibration of grief, but to, instead, consciously train our minds to focus on the future and not dwell in the past. Each of us has a destiny to fulfill, and we have got to get on with it. Moving on doesn't mean we will forget our son; it means we are honoring him and his memory by serving our purpose by helping others.

And although well-meaning, before you utter something stupid like, "Oh, God just needed another flower for his garden", to someone who has suffered a loss, please refrain. It only makes us want to punch you in the neck.

Judy is one of my heroes, because of her strong will, resilient spirit, and heart of servitude. In most of the instances of loss in her life, Judy was aware of the battle forthcoming. Following her beloved husband Gerry's example, Judy learned to join the battle of cancer with her loved ones, fight the feelings of fear, uncertainty, and hopelessness, and call upon the Infinite Source of strength, courage, and faith to see her through the interrupted rhythm of Life.

"Pain is inevitable, suffering is a choice."

-Unknown

Those of us who have survived the crisis of losing a loved one can certainly identify with that certain measure of time that is needed to process a devastating loss, and come to terms with it. It takes a committed decision to resolve your mind, settle your spirit, and accept it, before you can move on with your life. *It does take time,* and, in my opinion, *no one* has the right to tell you *how long* it should take to move through the grieving process after losing a husband, a child, a parent, or sibling, or even your beloved dog! Just don't suffer too long. Allow the deep pools of courage within your soul to rise to the surface and give you the strength you never knew you had, to get through a loss you never wanted. Find your courage to live.

In the chronicles of loss, Judy and her family mourned the death-by-cancer of her brother, Gary, in the year 2000. The next year, her father, who had battled with cancer for years, survived a stroke, but was left unable to care for himself. Her dad eventually succumbed to a massive, fatal stroke in 2005. Judy and her daughter, Amy, now shared a home with Judy's mother, and eventually, the three generations adjusted to the losses in their family. Judy grew very close to her mother after her father's death.

Eventually, finding the courage to open her heart to romantic love, Judy felt herself attracted to a very nice man whom the family was acquainted with for many years. Gerry and his dog, Snickers, had just moved into the family's house as boarders, but soon Gerry's quiet strength, generous nature, and love of travel and adventure won him a special place in Judy's heart. The two of them spent all their waking moments together, discovered how much they had in common, enjoyed traveling together, and very soon these soulmates were madly in love and planning their wedding.

On a magical October day, on a sparkling beach in Maui, Gerry and Judy exchanged vows and kisses while their families cheered and the waves applauded against the rocky shore. The lively celebration was slightly saddened by the unfortunate absence of Judy's mother, and their concern for her fatigue and recent weight loss. The family trusted that the doctors back home would soon have some answers. Mom, too ill to travel, put on a brave face, stayed home to rest, and took care of Snickers, who was now the family pet.

Within a few months, in the spring of 2008, Judy's mother was finally diagnosed with Stage IV lung cancer. In shock, the newlyweds were faced with taking the bulk of her mother's care upon themselves, running her to appointments, arranging her constant care, her meals, and staying close to her bedside as she deteriorated. My eyes watered as I read the complete, incredible accounting in Judy's book. In 2008, my family had also given care and stood by feeling helpless, as my beloved mother-in-law succumbed to inoperable pancreatic cancer, passing away within a month of Judy's mother, in the fall of that same year.

As hard as it is to process grief, you have to keep going, and that is just what Judy did, focusing on her job, and the part-time work she enjoyed in the literary world of her sister, Peggy McColl. However, by spring of 2009, she was laid off from her 15 year-long job. Scared, and still missing her mom terribly, this uncertainty was the last thing she needed in her life. Judy summoned her courage, once again, and at the suggestion and encouragement of her sister, Peggy, she optimistically trademarked her own company's name, Hasmark Services, and went to work!

"Everything is going to be okay"

~ Judy O'Beirn

Within weeks of starting over, Judy and her family's incomprehensible losses would begin to stack, one upon another, leaving her in an overload of grief, and a compounded crippling of all of the emotions that come with caregiving, disease, and tragic loss.

Their beloved Cockapoo, Snickers, suddenly became uncharacteristically sick. Very sick.

Cancer. Freaking, all-dogs-go-to-heaven, cancer. "LOW BLOW!", I want to scream out. I'm sure that thought crossed Judy's mind as well.

Sadly, he was gone within the month. And actually, there are many supporting stories of pets, especially dogs, who often take on the frequency of their owner, the illness or disease of their master. Whatever the cause, if you have ever lost a beloved pet who is like a member of the family, then you understand how that stabbing pain in your heart makes your knees weak, and your stomach churn. Fused with the recent loss of her mother, Judy was overwhelmed by the sadness of it all. To get through it, she chose to focus on all the good in her life, determined to move forward, with her "everything is going to be okay" mantra, and redirecting her energies on her new company, on her beautiful life with Gerry, and their traveling adventures together.

But, by the winter of 2010, the sequence of grieving suddenly continued, when they received an alarming phone call concerning Gerry's sister, Evelyn. She had just had a heart attack. She survived that battle, but lost the war; tests revealed horrifying results: Stage IV lung cancer. Beautiful Evelyn was gone within a week! Gerry, the rock of strength for the family, repeated the mantra, assuring everyone that they were going to be okay.

As the family reeled with shock and grief, during the weeks to follow, Gerry's other sister, Marlene, often mentioned the fatigue she was feeling. Her state of grief was suspected as the cause, but other symptoms developed, and by August, she was diagnosed with, you guessed it, cancer. Stage IV lung cancer. Unbelievable.

Gerry doted on his sister, determined to spend as much time with her as possible, assisting her, driving her, helping out around her house, taking care of legal matters, and offering his remarkable emotional support. Marlene fought hard, and even returned to work, despite the terminal disease. The family braced themselves with guarded hope.

That next winter, in 2011, Gerry himself had a heart attack while clearing their walkway of snow! Sister Marlene, even in her grim prognosis, came to see him immediately. After his surgery for a stent and a few weeks of bedrest, Gerry went back in for a regular, follow-up appointment. A routine test revealed a spot on his lung. And after many, many, more tests, poking, prodding, and biopsies, there was a diagnosis of a malignant cancer, Stage III. This was going to be a long battle.

Meanwhile, sister Marlene grew weaker and weaker. Gerry was at her side, spiritually strong and gentle, praying with her and holding her hand when she quietly slipped away. Another death. Another funeral. And another senseless loss of a beautiful life. Gerry was so physically weakened by his own cancer treatments that he struggled to make it through the service and reception. His quiet determination and strength fortified the family, and Judy's courage to walk this journey together surged.

Together, Gerry and Judy spent every waking minute battling the disease that plagued his body, while maintaining their hope, their passion for helping others, and their love for one another. It was a roller-coaster of appointments, tests, optimism, biopsies, waiting, anxiety, more tests, surgeries, more appointments, and endless caregiving that took its toll physically, mentally, and emotionally. Judy's nerves were completely shot with exhaustion and worry, ping-ponging between hope and despair, as the likelihood of Gerry's survival diminished.

Gerry decided to take what would be his last, adventurous trip with Judy to Florida. Away from hospitals, doctors, and appointments, he chose to focus on and enjoy the time he had left with his family. He made the most out of every day, while Judy held on with, "everything is going to be okay".

Meanwhile, Judy's daughter, Amy, was suddenly an angel of mercy for her best friend, who was just diagnosed with cancer. Mother and daughter, both consumed and isolated by the same experiences as a caregiver, felt the unexpected pain and frustration of not being able to help one another through this most difficult time. Judy would later reveal a mother's heart to me, with a poignant statement:

"So, it's not just me that I'm dealing with... I have my *daughter* going through this!"

Judy's distress at not being able to fully share her daughter's burden resonated with me. Living three hours away from our daughter, I found myself unable to be with our daughter, Leah, when she suddenly needed an emergency C-section. I was pacing outside of an E.R. 200 miles away, anxiously waiting for my husband, her dad, to come out of surgery to remove road shrapnel that was torpedoed into his leg while we were out riding motorcycles! I felt completely isolated, anxious, frustrated, helpless... aaaaand my cell-phone battery was dying.

"The apple doesn't fall far from the tree"
~ German Proverb

What transpired during Judy and Amy's experience was a stronger mother-daughter bond between them, as both courageous women gave selflessly to support the ones they loved, and offered moral support to each other, with advice, resources, information, answers, directions, and understanding.

Both of these strong women have a warrior-like passion for helping other people who have been affected by cancer.

Near the end of Gerry's courageous battle, Judy thought about writing a book, consumed by a driving need to do something for other families, to help them learn about caring for a loved one with cancer. She had become an expert on caregiving, and wanted to help others who get swept in by the whirlwinds of this greedy disease. She had the book cover designed in Gerry's favorite color of green, and was able to show it to him, before he slipped away in the cool, quiet hours of an April dawn.

I've mourned that I didn't get to know Gerry, personally. He was a great guy, judging his character by the way he lived his life with beautiful Judy, and by the stories she has shared about him. He was unselfish, and served others to the best of his ability. These two lovebirds were destined to be together, and Judy is blessed to have not only known him, but to have been the love of his life. Gerry was blessed to have married a woman of valor, a woman of courage. She has honored his memory by creating books, programs, and fundraisers with the intention of guiding others who have experienced loss to a peaceful place in their lives. Amy has joined her.

Judy is healing. It has been many years now, since Gerry passed; she misses him, but she's strong. She is determined to get up and have the courage to Live each day. She shares her incredible story with others, not for wanting to dwell on all the deaths, but to emphasize the magnitude of how quickly it all transpired. Judy knows in her spirit that a person can go through extreme challenges that would seemingly put them down to their knees, and yet, not only survive, but thrive.

There is a light at the end of the tunnel, and the light is

within you. Summon the courage within you, even when you don't think you have any, and it will get you through the dark, scary times. If Judy can do it, and I can do it, we know you can do it, and we are here to help you.

"Though I walk through the valley of the shadow of death..."

~ Psalms 23

It says, "walk THROUGH"... not stand in it. Do your grieving, and in time, learn to channel that energy into something positive for someone else; change your focus, and you'll change your life.

For more information, go to UnwaveringStrength.com

THREE

THE STORMS OF LIFE

In 2008, according to history, the Atlantic Hurricane Season was one of the most disastrous periods on record. It included 16 named storms and eight hurricanes, *five* of which were ranked as Category 3 or higher. These are considered *major* hurricanes because of their potential for significant loss of life and damage. The 2008 season caused over 1,000 deaths and nearly 50 Billion US Dollars in damages. Hurricane Ike, in particular, was one of the costliest storms in US history, and the costliest storm to ever ravage Cuba. Causing 38 Billion dollars in damage, Ike left a trail of devastation across Haiti, Cuba, and Texas. Due to its immense size, it affected places like the Bahamas, Turks and Caicos, Cayman Islands, and caused flooding and damages all along the Gulf Coast Region of Texas, Louisiana, Mississippi, and Florida. The search and rescue efforts after Ike were the largest in Texas history, up to that date. This was a time of devastation, a time for courage.

During this era, my husband, Chris, and I lived in Clear Lake City, a Southeastern annex of Houston. For over 30 years, we served the Gulf Coast area as Insurance Professionals. Even as seasoned veterans in the industry though, hurricane season always brought a tightening in my gut from day one until the end of November when the season ended. *This* season in 2008 had most everyone along the Gulf Coast Region on edge.

Historical accounts show Hurricane Ike began forming on Sept 1st and quickly strengthened; it intensified into a massive, Category 4 storm, with sustained winds of 145 MPH. People began stockpiling non-perishables, bottled water, batteries, generators, sandbags, boarding materials, and more. Grocery shelves were picked clean by panicked shoppers, long lines formed at gas pumps, evacuation plans discussed. There had been a close watch on Ike for nearly two weeks, witnessing its path of death and massive destruction via news reports. Many were praying it would dissipate before making landfall in our Gulf of Mexico. Now, we were looking down the barrel of this high velocity howitzer, and it was aimed straight at our Texas coastline. It was a sickening feeling, adding to the already excessive stress present in my and Chris' lives.

Considered part of the Bay Area, Clear Lake is just 30 miles inland from the coastal island of Galveston. Most all of our family and friends lived nearby. Earlier in 2008, anxiety had mounted within our family, as my beloved mother-in-law suffered with terminal, pancreatic cancer. Our oldest son, Eric, was at a residential facility, grinding out a long stint in rehab from substance abuse. On the homeowner's front, we were soon to be included among the casualties of the Mortgage Crisis of 2008. In our business lives, the insurance company we represented was renegotiating our contract again, and our agency had a client who was creating havoc with our bookkeeping. There was *much* to be concerned about and Hurricane Ike multiplied the worries and concerns, ten-fold.

On September 12th, the Texas Department of Insurance issued a Memorandum, a notice that states the official cut-off period of binding new business or increasing coverages once a storm enters the Gulf of Mexico. Those of us in the industry *knew*. Ike was over the line. This thing was coming. We closed the books, secured records, and prepared our offices. Chris and I sent our employees home. We took time to pull furniture away from the floor-to-ceiling, plate-glass windows, covered computers, and packed important files and documents for transport. Chris drove around the evacuated town where our office was located and inspected commercial buildings to verify the properties were secured.

We both took our oath as insurance agents very seriously. We chose to stay in town this time, as others evacuated, so we could serve our clients when the claims needed filing after the storm. We had ridden out many storms and hurricanes since living in Houston for over 25 years; we had evacuated for a few of them, experienced the fears, the frustrations, and traffic jams. We had stayed for other storms and experienced the fears, the flooding, and lack of utilities. We were now taking a calculated risk in choosing to ride out *this* hurricane.

Having done everything possible to take care of our agency and our clients, we closed the doors to our top floor offices, not knowing if there would be a roof or anything left when we returned. We made our way home through ominous winds, threatening skies darkened with heavy rains, a trunk full of documents, supplies, paper claim forms, and the heart-pounding feelings of dread and determination. It was time to prepare our own home for the hit, time to gather the family together, batten down the hatches, and "hunker down", as the news and weather guys like to say. This is when you know, things will never be the same.

Our two-story, brick home was strongly built, with extra hurricane straps and studs, and additional, above grade nails in the composite roofing. It was located at the high end of our neighborhood, and having never flooded in ten years, we felt relatively secure. We canvased our property and the deserted neighborhood for debris and loose items that might become projectiles. We made a mental note of the trampoline in the neighbor's yard. Once an agent, always an agent, inspecting for liabilities and accessing risk.

Thirty miles away, the historical City of Galveston on the island had been under Mandatory Evacuation for days. Port of Galveston, established in 1825, is an historical, Victorian, coastal resort town. She has stood as a sparkling jewel on the coastline, home to six historic districts, containing one of the largest and historically significant collections of 19th century buildings in the United States, with over 60 structures listed in the National Register of Historic Places. A favorite weekend getaway for so many, she has always been one of our favorite places to go, to breathe in the fresh ocean air, to feel the thundering waves on the sandy beaches, and listen to seagulls and laughter mingle in the sunshine. With a mindset of restoration, Galveston offers opportunity for growth and expansion for personal and commercial development. Whether one spends a day or goes on a weekend escape from the big city, a leisurely stroll down The Strand, a gaze at the Victorian Homes, a cruise down the Seawall, or a ride on the ferry boat, Galveston extends an invitation as a retreat to her visitors, an escape from the daily routine.

Now, as Hurricane Ike converged on the Texas coastline, Galveston was being pounded mercilessly by high winds, towering waves, and devastating flood waters. Thousands of homes and businesses were being impacted. Sentinel trees were being uprooted, some of them over 100 years old; historical Live Oaks, now driven by the winds, like torpedoes smashing into structures. The storm surge was scouring away beaches, eroding away roads, and erasing homesteads. Lives were in jeopardy; humans trapped in their homes, livestock with no high ground for refuge, and terrified birds and wildlife. Galveston was being ravaged like she had not seen since her demolishment by the deadliest hurricane in US history, the famous Storm of 1900.

Mick Petersen, a flight attendant by profession, had been living in Galveston for several years. He enjoyed the beach life, and all that the historic city offered, when he wasn't traveling with his career. Mick had also invested in real estate properties there, and the responsibilities and finances, as such. Galveston had seemingly never fully recovered to her former glory prior to the Storm of 1900. Like many others though, Mick saw her potential, and he had made it a mission to improve this little corner of the world.

The apartments and properties that he bought were cheap rentals, occupied by drug dealers and addicts, prostitutes and thieves. Mick courageously evicted these undesirable tenants, then made the investment and improvements necessary to attract a clientele who would take pride in their dwelling place. It had been a long and arduous journey filled with much difficulty, but now Mick was seeing the light at the end of a very long tunnel of renovations, contractors, and financial challenges. His spirits were soaring as he crossed over the Galveston Causeway Bridge towards the mainland, heading for the airport on his next assignment.

Mick was working as an attendant on a flight to Mexico City when Hurricane Ike turned its fury towards Galveston, Texas. All flights were cancelled as the Gulf Coast Region braced itself for the tempest storm. Stranded in Mexico with nowhere to go, Mick's usual cheerfulness began to evaporate as he thought pensively about his life. He was single, juggling a full-time career along with the responsibilities of his property and he was in the crosshairs of financial ruin caused by the Mortgage Crisis. As Hurricane Ike bore down on the Texas coastline, and realizing his properties' exposure and the seemingly insurmountable debt he was about to incur, Mick sank into deep despair. His home, his investments, and his life as he knew it, were going to be forever changed. It was overwhelming. In the dark hours of the morning of Sept 13th, as the catastrophic storm was making landfall, Mick sat alone in his hotel room, crestfallen. He journaled his anguish in three words, "All is lost".

Hurricane Ike raged on through the night, smashing houses, shredding historic piers and buildings, and pushing boats and debris ashore in Galveston. Fires raged, before the 19-foot tidal surge drowned them out and swept away the structures. The surge flooded thousands of homes, trapping unfortunate souls who couldn't evacuate in time. Sadly, 37 souls were later confirmed lost, with hundreds still missing to this day.

Farther inland, Ike crippled Houston with high winds and rain, blowing out skyscraper windows, stripping rooftops, toppling trees, and knocking out the electrical services to over four million people. Rising water flooded the streets and buildings in this Bayou City, but nothing seemed quite as devastating as what Galveston was experiencing. It was sickening to see the news reports before the electricity went out. Galveston was uninhabitable. She was drowning.

Thirty miles inland, our home stood solid, but eventually, the roof gave way to the high winds. Wind driven rain seeped into the attic, soaking the insulation and leaking through the boards until the sheet-rock ceilings came crashing down around our ears. Howling wind beat against the back door, as both upstairs and down, and around windows and doors, the rain seeped in. Squinting in the darkness, we took turns braving the gale forces to assess the rising water and airborne debris. There is something almost mesmeric about nature's wrath that lures man into gazing at it in disbelief and wonder.

Our grown kids and first grandchild were gathered with us at our house. Our son Eric was visiting home from rehab for the first time that weekend. Internally concerned, as parents we put on a brave face and assured them all of our safety. Everyone chipped in to clean up the soggy mess, move furniture, and pull back wet carpets. We set out pots to catch the leaks, window sills were lined with towels, and we all took turns checking the structure of the house. The winds howled until dawn. The sunrise on September 13th revealed the incredible shredding of roofs and trees, downed fences, and the neighbor's trampoline twisted like abstract artwork in their yard. The eye of the storm had passed; we were safe, but it was going to be a long recovery for us and for everyone else in the destructive pathway of Ike.

Mick was finally able to return to Galveston, holding very little hope for the future. The island was under curfew, with a limited return of residents. His heart sank as he picked his way through miles of wreckage and debris along Interstate 45. The Gulf Freeway was an obstacle course filed with drifts of yachts and sailboats lying in piles like forgotten toys tossed aside in an epic tantrum. Smashed vessels and the rubble of thousands of homes now littering the flooded roadways. As he topped the Causeway Bridge over the Gulf Intracoastal Waterway, the horrendous devastation was visible for as far as one could see. Once on the island, he saw overturned cars lying in giant mud puddles and homes reduced to kindling. Graves were unearthed, coffins lay askew. Landmarks, trees, and street signs were eradicated. There was no electricity, no clean water, and no food, and very little hope in this fetid wasteland.

Mick arrived to find that his own properties were in ruins. After four feet of water and five days of sweltering heat, the stench was unbearable. The foul air was swarming with mosquitos, sewage had backed up into the standing water in the streets, and mold permeated everything. Overturned refrigerators festered with rotting food. Critters and cockroaches scattered from under waterlogged couches. Snakes and rusty nails threatened in the murkiness. Gathering his courage, Mick rolled up his sleeves, and got to work.

Cut to 2018. Nearly ten years after that devastating year changed the trajectory of my life and career, I was in Ottawa, Canada, attending a writer's event hosted by my mentor, Peggy McColl. One morning before the meeting began, I sat in the empty room and reflected; a lot had transpired in my life during the past decade. My mother-in-law had succumbed to cancer within two months of Hurricane Ike. That cursed storm and the Mortgage Crisis of 2008 had brought Chris and me to our financial knees. Challenged by an eight figure lawsuit which was filed after Ike against our agency and the insurance companies we represented, our lives were consumed with anxiety for 18 months during the proceedings.

The damage had been done to our spirits. Not having the skill sets back then to handle the stress of all of this, it manifested itself in my body as a Takotsubo cardiomyopathy. The debilitating "broken-heart syndrome" episode put me in I.C.U. for three days. Eventually, I recovered, but I never returned to insurance again; my heart just wasn't in it anymore, literally and figuratively. We sold our agency and moved inland to Central Texas to begin anew.

Now, as I sat in peace in the gathering space of our event, I closed my eyes and meditated on how I had gotten through all of those events. I had faced my fears. I weathered through the storms that Life blew my way. No, it wasn't easy; in fact, these traumatic events *sucked*. But, I didn't give up. *We* didn't give up. Chris and I had begun to study personal development. I read voraciously (and still do). We began attending seminars, events, and courses, gaining knowledge and applying it to our lives, growing in wisdom through our experiences. By the time the worst tragedy of all occurred – the death of our son Eric on November 13, 2015, my mastery of courage saw me through.

Quitting is not an option.

At the writer's event in Ottawa, we were all to take a turn making our presentation to the group. Realizing I was quivering with a bit of nervous energy, I summoned my courage and volunteered to speak first. It was my inaugural, live presentation of this sort and I was anxious to get started. The room was filled with so many beautiful people: my mentor, my friends and peers, a tribunal of good-hearted critiques. All of us had a sense of importance of the messages we wanted to share with this world. As I stepped forward, I looked confident enough, but I was shaking on the inside. I took a slow, deep breath and began.

That talk felt like the shortest 15 minutes in my career. I didn't gage the time correctly and came up short on the Revenue Plan portion of my presentation. It really peeved me, because I wanted to ace that talk! I returned to my seat; in my head the score was Storytelling, ten, Business Plan, zero. Go, me. I mentally berated myself for the rest of the day, as I otherwise gave my attention to the other wonderful presentations. Berated, that is, until the last person began his talk.

I sat listening intently as one of my favorite fiction authors gave his presentation to our elite circle. Handsome, with a boyish charm and an incredible, storytelling gift, Mick Petersen stood before our group, and referred back to where "it" all began for him – the devastation in 2008 that brought him "the dream" that forever changed his life.

Mick began his presentation with some background information. He recollected being stranded in a hotel in Mexico City. He had been full of despair as news of Hurricane Ike made headlines around the globe. His properties surely lost, he had contemplated the massive debt he had been handed from the storm, the Mortgage Crisis, and from his former partner. On the eve of September 13, 2008 as he drifted off to sleep in that lonely hotel room, Mick wondered what sort of glorious life he might live once all the crap ahead had been dealt with. Without realizing he was employing courage, he allowed himself the opportunity to dream about a better life. He dared to wonder, "what do I want? What do I REALLY want?"

"In the middle of the night, I gasped awake from the most glorious dream. In it, I had met Stella."

Mick, of course, was referring to the main character in his #1 Best Seller, *Stella and the Timekeepers*. Over the course of the next three years, Mick had allowed himself to wander in the fertile playground of his imagination. Stella became his tour guide, as he learned more and more of the three realms that comprised this imagined world. Mick's dreaming transported him from the difficulties of his "real" life, to a place of respite, calm, and tranquility. It was a world of curiosity and abundance. Along the way, a better path revealed itself to Mick, and his external world transformed into betterment.

Now, some ten years in the creating, today Mick was presenting to us "The 3 Realms" of his Stella trilogy. We all felt the magic of his amazing, storytelling abilities. As Mick spoke, I was astonished when I realized that the *same*, calamitous hurricane in 2008, and the *same* Mortgage Crisis, had changed the course of *both* of our lives. And now, here we were as fellow authors, in Ottawa, Canada, with the same mentor, at the same convocation, presenting on the same day. More importantly, we were friends! You can't make this stuff up.

SACRED SPACE

I couldn't help but smile as Mick read a passage to us from a favorite book. The slide presentation mechanics had hiccups, so he had no big screen media slides, but he didn't let that faze him. His presentation was stronger and more meaningful because it came from his soul. He was animated, articulate, and spoke, at times, in childlike wonderment of his own incredible journey. I truly felt we were all bound together in this sacred space, sharing our dreams, stating our business plans, and opening our hearts. This space was pure and authentic. I was safe to seemingly fail among these like-minded authors, my like-hearted friends. I released my negative feelings of defeat and chose to embrace the good stuff I had presented; I'd learn from the mistakes I made during my talk. *Next time I will be better*, I declared inwardly, as I grinned at my literary fairy. His words were like sparkling dust particles of encouragement on my Spirit.

Mick went on to share his story, passionately stating that he had chosen not to give up and file bankruptcy after Hurricane Ike, but had mustered through his financial challenge, worked hard and paid off a ninety-thousand-dollar debt he had incurred. I knew of the tremendous courage to go through the challenges that Hurricane Ike brought, and I sensed a certain pride in his overcoming the outstanding debt, *and* in record time, he had emphasized.

Then, in a flash, I had rapid-fire thoughts: hey, wait a minute… just because someone files for bankruptcy doesn't mean they have given up! My husband and I had to file for bankruptcy, and we weren't giving up; we had very little other choice! Our mortgagee had royally screwed up our mortgage, putting us in jeopardy of losing our home. At the advice of our attorney, we filed for reorganization. The suggestion was nauseating, but it saved our property. A consolidation was made, a payment plan set up, and we paid off the debt.

My next thought was of what Bob Proctor had once taught during an event: *being offended is a choice*. It is a feeling, an emotion. We must set a goal of developing the ability to control and direct our feelings and emotions. I know that developing the virtue of courage supports that goal. When you know you should act or feel a certain way, the Right way, and it may even bother you to "have to be the grownup", *that is when your developed courage comes into play*.

I sat beaming at Mick and at myself as I made a conscious decision not to be offended by his remark. Rapidly, the thoughts went through my mind; it took courage for *both* of us to make our decisions. We had *both* made sacrifices, paid our debts, and, along the way, discovered our true destinies. We had each taken a different path, yet both paths led us to *today*, together, in this elite circle, into this sacred space.

It takes courage to let go of pettiness, negative thoughts, and "peevement", if you will. At times we may think we are *entitled* to feel the negative emotions that we are hosting, like anger, resentment, and *being offended*. But, we always have a choice. The more you exercise this most important virtue called Courage, the stronger it becomes, the *stronger* you become, until being courageous in all parts of your life becomes second nature. It gets easier and easier to hold Right thoughts, make good choices and decisions, dispel fear, and take deliberate actions.

I relaxed. Confidently, I took a deep breath in, grateful for the journey. It hadn't been easy, but here I was. I breathed out. Here, I AM. Go, me.

For more information on Mick, go to
stellaandthetimekeepers.com

FOUR

THE STAGE OF LIFE

Most all of us go through life attempting to satisfy roles for which we have been seemingly cast, programed through the environmental conditioning to which we are subjected to, right from birth.

Our subconscious mind registers EVERYTHING, from the day we are born. We are the very DNA from our parents and ancestors. We act a certain way, have certain mannerisms, certain dispositions and personalities. Our environment forms our social understanding, our family roles, we receive gender cues, physical development and appearance conclusions, our school experiences, teachers, and peer groups, ethnicity, racial, and religious profiles, media, trauma, drama… it ALL shapes and forms our perception and attitude towards EVERY-THING, not the least of which is our own self-image, how we see ourselves.

As children we grow and mature, developing cognition around age six to seven years old. From birth we are subjected to other people's opinions, other people's rules and expectations about *who* we should be, *how* we should think and act, and *what* our destiny is to fulfill. And many of us are taught, "don't ask *why*". Everything from behavioral examples at home, our gradation in school, degrees, athletics, relationship rules, and parenting directives, to careers, work ethics, and income expectations, contributes to our "own" opinions, mindset and attitude. Worst of all, somewhere along the way, most people are also programed to accept failure as "it just wasn't meant to be", and settle for being a typecast actor in their own play.

And yet, WE ARE EACH RESPONSIBLE FOR OUR OWN CHOICES, ACTIONS, AND RESULTS.

We are all actors, performing roles based on ideas that aren't even our own, futile walk-ons in the theater of Life. Many times, we are playing the supporting role in someone else's life, rarely endeavoring to star in the production of our *own* creation. Worst yet, sitting in an audience of adversity, we are pacified to critique and heckle others in this same, prosaic arena.

> *"You can play supporting roles to Fear your whole life.*
> *Is that what you want?"*

> ~ Stella Adler, Grande Dame of American Theater,
> legendary Acting Teacher

Being an insurance agent/broker was always my husband Chris' passion. His sales career started in 1979, soon after we were married. In the late 1980s, he convinced me to come to the office and team up with him, so as soon as our three children were in school full-time, I joined him. Being in sales and service was a new role for me, and out of my comfort zone. I pushed myself hard, studied, learned, and acted like an agent, but didn't really enjoy my role. Employed by a large, national insurance company, Chris was the Primary Agent, while they considered me "support staff". Chris was recognized and respected as one of the top agents in the State of Texas. I drew no salary or credit, but Chris was astute enough to call all of the commissions, awards, and acclaims ours, to help me realize my worth to the agency and to him. We were Team Bazzy, working on his dreams, visions, and ambitions.

Acting the part of the role I was now cast into, I eventually became really good at it. I made myself even more knowledgeable, dressed the part wearing suits to the office, and carried myself well in the role. I became our office manager and headed up the Personal lines of insurance, like auto, homeowners, flood, etcetera, while Chris was out in the field, working the Commercial and Life lines of products and coverages. We made a great professional team. A lot of times, that's what marriage is about – teamwork.

The next company that hired us recognized me as an equal, which felt good, and encouraged me to push my role and responsibilities even further. I assumed more authority, acting as both agent and owner of our business. I managed the office, built a staff, kept the books, oversaw our compliance with the State of Texas, did annual reviews, took care of public relations, advertising, licensing, sold and serviced policies, and made friends out of customers. I began to really enjoy my career, although it was all *highly* stressful on me.

Chris and I went through a decade of tumultuous years, which was an aggregation of traumas that covered so many areas of our lives. Our insurance careers were besieged with stress and challenges; we had a serious automobile accident, which resulted in cumulative hospital bills and subsequent bankruptcy; there were IRS issues, hurricanes, damages and lawsuits, and the terrible loss of Chris' mom to cancer. Throughout the entire period, our family suffered the incredible, stressful impact of having a son and brother who was a substance abuser. Eric was in and out of rehabs, trouble with the law, and strife. It seemed like this whole dark tunnel of tribulation would never end.

I didn't think about courage during this time. I just did what had to be done and struggled through the chaos. Fact is, my lack of proper thinking and underdeveloped higher faculties resulted in *severe stress*, which put me in the I.C.U. with a Takotsubo cardiomyopathy attack, also known as broken-heart syndrome. I just called it a heart-fart. Yeah, me.

I eventually recovered, and Chris and I made some radical decisions. We sold our agency, put the house on the market, and we moved back to my hometown of San Antonio. I retired from the insurance industry. After 30 years of professional service, I was out. It had never been my chosen vocation, even if I *was* great at it. My heart, literally and figuratively, just wasn't in it anymore.

Chris took on a new venture, and eventually, we recovered our financial losses, and were up and running again. I say "we"; it was really Chris, and his entrepreneurial spirit, that got the money flowing once again. I hibernated in our little condo, decompressed, and sort of withdrew from all social activities. I had no plans, no goals, and no idea what I wanted to do. I dabbled in my writing, did research for a book; I painted, created jewelry, and gardened. I felt a sort of emptiness, once the "new" wore off as a character of retirement. I was bored; I felt incomplete. At first, I relished my unemployment, but soon I felt dissatisfied. Something gnawed at my gut. I should be doing *something*, but what?

In April of 2016, Chris and I attended Proctor Gallagher Institute's Matrixx event in Toronto, Canada. Chris had his game plan, and I went along because we do almost everything together. Over the past two years, we had been on a journey of self-awareness and personal growth, had attended Tony Robbins' Mastery University, and now we were studying with Bob Proctor. I knew I was *supposed* to be at Matrixx; I just had no idea *why* I was there.

"Restlessness is discontent – and discontent is the first necessity of progress. Show me a thoroughly satisfied man –

and I will show you a failure."

~ Thomas Edison
The Diary and Sundry Observations of Thomas Alva Edison
(1948), p. 110.

When it comes to the internet, you can't swing a dead cat without hitting the word "paradigm". In fact, you can hit it over 87,200,000 times in under half a second, if the results meter is correct on Google. This word "paradigm" used to have an obscure, ambiguous definition in my mind, something I had never really studied or grasped the full meaning of. That is, until I met Bob.

The best definition and teaching I have ever heard comes from Bob Proctor, who is widely regarded as the world's foremost expert on the human mind; a master and teacher, who has worked in the area of mind potential for over 50 years. Bob Proctor teaches us that a paradigm is a mental programing in our subconscious mind, which has almost exclusive control over our habits. It is a collection of thoughts, beliefs, and conditioning; a multitude of habits, which control our behavior.

I participated in Matrixx with an open mind. Listening to Bob, I realized I was an actor; I had gone through my entire life, performing duties and obligations based on ideas that weren't even my own. I was a futile walk-on in a melodramatic role of existence. Thanks to Bob and his partner, Sandy Gallagher, I understood that I was one of those programed people that they were referring to. Talented and bright, but ignorant of how the Laws of the Universe operate, I had been a struggling student in school, an anxious people pleaser, and a ball-busting mom, because that was all I knew how to be.

Now as I sat in a room full of entrepreneurs, it seemed to me that everyone was either looking to improve an existing career, or kick-start a new one. I began to think, "So, what can *I* do? What can *I* create?" That nasty paradigm popped up its ugly head, taunting me. "What can *you* do? You're too old to start over. You're not pretty enough, skinny enough, you don't have a degree in anything, you're not an expert on anything. Who do you think you are?!" Then I came face to face with the unavoidable question that had been looming all week:

"What do you want; What do you really want?!"

My mind was reeling. We had a breakout session – a table talk – where the six participants at each table were to ask each other *the* question, "What do you want; What do you *really* want?" The answers needed to be concise and well defined. With limited time for this exercise, the final instruction was for the table to vote on who would start. My table voted for *me* to go first, much to my horror.

"GO!" came the command from the stage. The room erupted in excitement. My experience felt like my table pounced on me like a pack of hyenas! Overly excited and hyped, they all began to shout at once, unnerving me at my core. That paradigm of unworthiness was still kicking and screaming inside my head; *"Who do you think you are?"* It was now or never. I summoned my courage and blurted out what I had denied myself my entire life.

"I want to be an author."

The chaos that followed was overwhelming. Everyone excitedly spoke all at once, with so many questions, I couldn't clearly hear or understand any of them. The chaos at the table and my fear nearly had me in tears. "What have I done?!" The mediator calmed everyone down and came around to my side of the table for support. The most aggressive guy in our group slapped his hand on the table, drawing my attention. "Okay, what TYPE of author?" he demanded, as though I were on trial. I paused for only a couple of seconds, but that was too long for the anxious table of my enthusiastic peers. The clamor exploded as everyone began offering the suggestions of various genres of books, as if I didn't know my own dreams. Something inside me shifted. I'd had about enough of this crap. I sat up straight and squared my shoulders. Leaning forward towards my aggressor, I looked him straight in the eyes and stated firmly and matter-of-factly,

"*A New York Times Best Selling Author!*"

Well, that shut him up. In fact, it shut the whole table up.

Have you ever made such a bold statement, and then wondered what orifice it fell out of? Yeah, that was me at that moment. I thought, *well, I said it, so it's out there.* I had finally admitted out loud, to relative strangers, one of my deepest desires. My insides were shaking; my heart was pounding. This is no game. This is my *life!* And since I had already made this bold public statement, I decided, why not? *Why not me?!*

It is no coincidence that during that Matrixx event I met Peggy McColl. It was April 13th; exactly five months had passed since our son's death. I had seen Peggy on a couple of Proctor Gallagher Live feed events prior to attending in person and I had looked up her webpage to learn more about her. Peggy is a *New York Times* Best Selling Author and Internationally recognized speaker, author, and teacher. She is an expert in the area of goal achieving; she is an author's author. Now here she was, *in person*, speaking to our Matrixx class; I felt such a connection with her, and a deep desire to work with her. I didn't know how it would transpire, but I knew that I needed Peggy.

I made it my business to meet Peggy after she delivered her presentation about a new project she was hosting. The book project was titled *DESTINIES*; a collection of motivating stories from ordinary people who created extraordinary results. OMG. I just about fell off my chair. *I saw my destiny as an author.* I signed up immediately as a contributing author to her *Destinies* project. The book would later become a #1 Amazon Best Seller in several categories, including International Best Seller.

Through Peggy McColl and participating in her programs, I met my good friend and accountability partner, Colleen Aynn. Since we are both mentored by Peggy, we see one another on video chat calls and attend a lot of the same events together. She and I were talking one day about our experiences of reinvention, laughing as we shared our stories with one another. Colleen is bubbling with life, with sparkling eyes, a genuine smile, and has an infectious "let's do this" attitude. She is truly creative and has proven so in the last few years by re-creating herself and reinventing her passion for serving others.

Colleen has performed all over the world as a singer, actor, and dancer. She has been a professional actress since age ten; it was her *passion*, her *life*, and she loved, loved, loved it, up until she had a baby. At eight and a half months pregnant, she was doing a show, and loving it. Once she gave birth to her daughter, who was a "colicky mess", her self-confidence, self-worth, and sanity seemed to evaporate overnight. Colleen was used to walking onto a stage or entering a room with people applauding. Instead, now she had a baby who would just scream in her face, all day long. Colleen would sing to her, dance circles for her, speak in funny voices… and, nothing. The baby heckled back with screaming.

Colleen was ragged, handing off the wailing infant to her husband, Bruno, when he came home at night. He is a doctor and, at the time, he worked 10 to 12 hour shifts. She had been "a performer and worked long hours in the theater. Their schedule had worked when it was just the two of them, but *now* there was this third, little person disrupting their ten-year marriage, routine, and emotions. She would hand off the baby, go stand in the shower, and cry. Her solitude with an inconsolable, screaming baby 12-14 hours a day, was taking its toll on her psyche. Mommie was a mess. She began going to therapy; she and her husband attended marriage counseling. She loved their daughter but felt herself getting lost in the role she now was now cast into.

Colleen had planned to take a year off from performing after she gave birth; however, when their daughter was about seven months old, Colleen received a phone call offering her a job opportunity which she jumped at; she didn't care what the role was or how much it paid, the answer was yes, Yes, YES!! For the next few months, she tried to bring the baby with her to the theater; she brought a nanny, then her mother, even her husband, when he wasn't on call. Nothing worked. She finally arranged for childcare at their home, while she performed.

One day her husband texted her photos of him and their daughter in the pool together. Colleen went back stage and burst into tears. Sobbing, she asked herself, "*WHY am I doing this?!*" Soul-searching, she bemoaned, "I used to love this. This is what I *lived* for, and now what I live for is 300 kilometers away… *what am I doing!?*" She knew she had to change her life. She finished her contract with the company and returned to become a stay-at-home mommy.

The only problem was, she felt that she wasn't very good at being a stay-at-home mommy. She didn't fit in with the "mom groups"; she changed what seemed like a hundred diapers a day, she wasn't a very good cook; in fact, she didn't like to cook. She felt trapped. Again, she found herself asking, "What am I going to do with my life?" She didn't want to perform because she wanted to be with her family; she didn't want to be with her family *this* much, because it was *too much*. She found herself in a weird place that I would bet a lot of new moms find themselves in, asking, "Now what?"

I'd also be willing to bet that lots of moms, myself included, have felt guilty for not feeling completely fulfilled with staying home with their child or children. Colleen certainly felt guilty. She questioned, "*Why* aren't I completely satisfied with just being a mom, and having a healthy kid? I have a beautiful house, nice cars, a great husband, the "perfect life" – and I don't feel satisfied or complete". She was miserable. So, now what?

Colleen was asking the right questions and being honest with herself. She didn't know why she wasn't happy… she *wanted* to be happy and satisfied, but this wasn't something she could pretend she was. *Acting* was her lifelong profession, yet she couldn't *act* happy. What was wrong? She had always loved life and looked forward to getting up each morning to go to work. It didn't even feel like "work" because she was so passionate about her calling. Now, the daily numbing of changing diapers, fixing meals, doing laundry and chores, and all to the tune of a crying baby, was driving her attitude into the dumpster. She wasn't her same, happy, life-loving character. She'd become, in her words, bitchy.

We all need to ask questions and examine our lives. If something doesn't feel right, then instead of stuffing the feelings, becoming angry or depressed, taking medications or turning to destructive alternatives, get some help! Colleen went to a lot of therapy for depression, for the feelings of being lost, trapped, and not knowing what to do. She did not give up her search for the answers.

"I can't do this. I don't like my life – and that's awful – that's a crappy realization, 'I don't like my life', and I'm only 35."

~ Colleen Aynn

Two things happened that turned Colleen away from depression and towards the happy life she now lives. One happened when she had returned to the theater when her daughter was seven months old. Colleen had played the part of June Carter Cash in a show. During the scene when Colleen portrayed June "writing lyrics" for a song, Colleen sat on the stage and doodled on a pad of paper. The subconscious doodling took the form of little characters. During each performance, she would doodle these little faces, naming them, and assigning character traits to each one.

Later, she'd take herself out to breakfast, and draw them out. Eventually, she began hearing their stories in her head, so she wrote the stories down. They sounded like children's books to her. She didn't know at the time, but these characters would later turn into the *Feeling Friends* children's books series that have made her an International Best Selling Author.

The second thing that happened was when she returned home one night and found her husband reading a book about panic attacks. She thought, *What? Holy crap, what's going on?!* He said that he had an upcoming presentation and was really stressed about it. Colleen confidently offered with a smile, "Oh, I can help you with *that*", to which he poo-foo'd away. He dismissed her offer with a remark, "You're not going to know what it's about. It's all medical stuff". She replied cheerfully, "I don't care *what* it's about. It doesn't matter; I can help you with the presentation side of it".

Her husband put her off for six months, until finally, he was so stressed out he gave in one day. He succumbed in the living room and eked out his request for help. "Fine... just do that thing you do... it's not going to work, but, go ahead... do your thing". Ten minutes into her "thing" and he was fully engaged. "Holy crap, why don't they teach us this stuff?!" Doctors (and other professionals) receive no training in the area of presentations, speeches, or talks that they must make on a regular basis. How was he supposed to get up in front of hundreds of colleagues and peers (one of the hardest audiences), with no training?

So, Colleen helped him, because that's what we do when we love someone. People started noticing his presentations were getting better and better. He answered their inquiries about his process by referring to his wife who coached him. Before long, Colleen was being approached by her husband's colleagues with questions. Here were these curious intellectuals trying to connect with an artist. "Sooo, you're an actress? And, you, uh, helped your husband? Would you, uh, like, help *us*?"

Colleen agreed, wholeheartedly. She built a presentation based on the attendees' needs and created her first workshop for the one of the departments in the hospital. THEN she realized who would be attending; all of the bigwigs would be there She freaked out! Her paradigm screamed, "What have you done, *NOW!?!*" This was a terrible idea! She had taught throughout her entire career; taught piano lessons at age 14, gave acting lessons at age 18, and coached voice at the age of 24. The teaching part didn't make her nervous. It was the fear of attempting to teach this art form to a room full of intellectuals – doctors! – that made her nervous. She felt so intimidated, with disempowering thoughts like, "How can lil ol' me, an actress, go in and teach *them*? What are you doing? Why would you do this? Terrible idea. *Who do you think you are?*"

She had never been scared of anything before in her life. She had performed on stage since she was a very young child, something that would terrify most adults. She was raised in the limelight and practically glowed in the dark with confidence. Now she had to dig deep for the courage to push through her terror and teach this class. A courage that she hadn't needed to fully develop until now.

"Don't be afraid of your fears. They're not there to scare you. They're there to let you know that something is worth it."

~ *C. JoyBell C.*

Colleen gave one of the best performances of her life. The curtain calls came from department after department throughout the hospital. Word of mouth promoted this newfound teaching and coaching until one day, she was cast to perform for a Broadway Show, otherwise known as the Cardiac Surgeons Department. Again, the paradigm coughed up the doubt and the negative questions in her head. "What the hell am I doing?!" echoed in her mind, but she pushed through, using her newfound courage.

During this process of reinventing herself, Colleen discovered the answers to "Who am I?" She began reading and studying. She came across a children's book and she got the idea to turn this material into a play and tour it around all of the schools. The paradigm was waiting to push that idea aside; "Who do you think you are? You can't do this! Who are you, that he's going to want *you* to turn his book into a play?" She set the idea aside.

Within a couple of weeks, Bob Proctor popped up on an ad. Suddenly, there was this beautiful message making a point, "Why *not* you?" That simple question resonated with Colleen to the point of tears. Sobbing, she proclaimed out loud, "Damn right, why *not* me!" She emailed the author with her idea. The response was immediate: the idea was loved! The author asked for final approval of the script and encouraged her to *go for it!* Once again, terrified and elated, Colleen began studying the works of Bob Proctor and the methods he teaches. She watched his videos persistently, in order to build up her courage.

> *"I would watch a Bob video, do something big,*
> *hit send, then want to throw up."*
>
> ~ Colleen Aynn

This was her process that she repeated over and over, as she submitted a script, talked to literary agents in New York, and negotiated with lawyers. Clueless as to what she was doing, she was taking action anyway. Finally, she decided that if she had gotten this far by watching his videos, she needed to meet Bob Proctor in person. She chose an event in her hometown of Toronto, the Matrixx, and going with her strong gut feeling, insisted on her husband attending with her. Always follow your Knowing.

While at Matrixx, Bob asked from the stage, "Who here has written a book?" Colleen sat quietly, smiling, glancing around at the others in the room. She didn't even consider the question. She suddenly heard a hissing and loud whisper from behind. "Colleen, raise your hand! Colleeeeen, raise your hand!" It was her hubby, three tables behind her. She weakly raised her hand halfway up, thinking, "Well, it's just a kids' book. Oh, I haven't done anything with it. I don't think he's talking about me." (That paradigm should be named Chatty Cathy and have a zipper on her mouth!).

Bob turned and looked right at Colleen, and matter-of-factly told her, "Publish your book!" Her response was, "Well, I am a singer. I don't know how to do that". Bob pointed out Peggy McColl and told Colleen, "Go see Peggy and say 'hi'; she knows what she's doing". Suddenly, it made sense. Everything clicked. OMG.

Colleen realized that Bob Proctor was teaching acting. Act like the person you want to be. "I've been acting on stage, why am I not acting in my life? I have no problem being center stage in a theater, so *why am I not center stage in my own life?* OH, *that's done.*" Drawing a line in the imaginary sand, Colleen stepped away from entertaining the negative thoughts. She had lived her dream in the past; it was time to live her new dream NOW.

Colleen took back center stage. She got Peggy as her mentor, publishing her first book. Then three more books followed. She developed and now teaches courses; she is a coach, and is an encourager to all who know her. Colleen found the courage to say, "This is my *life*, and I can do whatever I set my mind to do!"

"Act as though I am, and I will be."

- Dr. Joseph Murphy

Colleen and I both realized that it was up to each of us to take our own life back and reinvent ourselves. We both refused to give up. Success is in loving your work, and it is never too late, and you are *never* too old or *too anything*, to take center stage in your own life.

I am amused by the serendipity of Colleen and my experiences at the Matrixx. The timing was just a few months apart from one another. The Matrixx event and our "Bob encounter" were paramount in both of our lives, and many others' lives. It was, to quote Bob and Sandy, a *Paradigm Shift*.

After our Matrixx event, at the end of the week, the class was invited to Bob and his wife Linda's home for a reception. My husband and I enjoyed the privilege of being in their home and the warm company of our classmates. I marveled at Bob's enormous library, being a bibliofreak myself. As we were all leaving their beautiful home, our event host was handing out a gift. Artistically crafted on linen, it was a beautiful reminder:

"Those who dream by day are cognizant of many things which escape those who dream only by night."

~ Edgar Allan Poe

I got so excited when I read the inscription! I had come across the quote recently and had written it in the front cover of my copy of Bob's book *The Art of Living*. I had brought the book with me to Toronto, hoping to get his autograph (it's one of my favorite books), but somehow left it in our hotel room. I was so enthusiastic about the "coincidence" of the quote, that I forgot my insecurities and went back to the porch where Bob was finishing his goodbyes. I waited my turn, then bubbled up my joyful discovery.

Bob looked at me with those thoughtful blue eyes of his and then asked, "So, where's the book?"

My insides deflated; so, I made light of the matter and responded with a joke. Hanging my head in mock shame, I said, "Forgive me, Father, for I have sinned". Chuckling, he grabbed my hand and dragged me quickly (in my high heels) through the entire house, through the backyard, past the pool, to where his office and recording studio are built. That man can walk *fast!* I followed him inside to his office. It was a bit like being in the inner sanctuary. Bob went to a drawer and took out a new copy of *The Art of Living*, and addressed it to me, with best wishes. I was ecstatic!

Then, Bob paused, as if listening to a whisper in his ear. He went back to another drawer and pulled out a beautiful hardback copy of *The Art of Acting*, by Stella Adler. My heart leaped! That book was on the top of my reading list! He thought for a second, and then signed it with a proclamation,

> *"Rachel, Make it happen.*
> *Bob Proctor"*

And here, I Am.

For information on Colleen's work, go to colleenaynn.com

FIVE

THE ANATOMY OF COURAGE

Several years ago, my husband and I stepped up our studies on personal growth by attending a Tony Robbins event called "Unleash the Power Within". It was life changing. I felt both challenged and victorious, and by the end of the event, my mind was blown and my voice was raspy from participation. Along with thousands of other attendees, I hoarsely shouted our new affirmation, "NOW, I AM THE VOICE". Truly, my life has never been the same since that first event.

It is an awesome feeling to be a part of something so huge, so positive, and so transformational in my own life and other people's lives. The friendships we have formed from these experiences will last a lifetime. As Chris and I completed the Mastery University series of events, we also found the spiritual need and personal reward in making a contribution; paying it forward. We have volunteered, and continue to do so, our time and energy as Crew members at various Tony Robbins events.

It was on one of my first Crewing experiences that I met Willard Barth. Willard serves on Crew as often as his busy schedule allows. I have witnessed him in the middle of the heat, swiftly maneuvering around burning coals, barking out orders to the Fire Team like a seasoned captain, and the next day, delivering a heartfelt presentation in the Crew room that brings inspiration, information, and transformation.

Willard Barth is a remarkable man. He is an International Business and Life Coach, Speaker, Best Selling Author, and a true friend to all those he meets. Willard is about giving back, and he serves his fellow humanity in his very special way. I have often observed him sitting with someone, holding a private consultation, offering guidance, encouragement, sharing his wisdom, and uplifting spirits. He is energetic, courageous, has an infectious smile, and a grateful, heartfelt passion for serving others.

And, he is the fastest man on crutches I have ever seen.

You see, when Willard was eight years old, he was diagnosed with bone cancer. Faced with making a decision to prolong his life, his mother summoned her courage and made the agonizing decision to have his leg amputated. There were no other treatment alternatives back in 1973. Cancer was considered a death sentence. She rose to the challenge, and forbade the doctor from telling young Willard, the family, or anyone else about the disease. She barred him from sharing the prognosis of a three to five-year window of life expectancy. She didn't want Willard living every day of his life thinking it was his last, nor to have people focusing on him in that way. Willard's mother made this courageous choice of keeping this pronouncement between the doctor and herself. She chose to focus on his *life*, and ignore the diagnosis of a 95-97% probability of cancer returning. She guarded her thoughts and vocabulary, and spoke positivity into Willard's mind. Growing up he never considered that every time he coughed, he could have caused his mother anxiety over his health. She must have developed tremendous courage, as she battled the concern for his delicate life, keeping the illness a secret unto herself.

"Courage is being scared to death, but saddling up anyway".

~ John Wayne

Willard reflects that his mother infused in him a sense that we must just *do* what needs to be done. Detached, Willard's biological father never intended to show up for a wedding to this young woman. It was 1965. Amid the opinions of those around her, the social stigma of being a single mother, the suggestions of getting rid of the pregnancy, giving up or abandoning her child, Willard's mother courageously chose to keep her baby. Against all odds, she worked three jobs to support herself, her mother, and her new son. Willard admiringly recalls that he never saw his mother miss a day of work. She mustered through sickness, poor weather, and incredible challenges, and showed up to do what needed to be done. He believes this was the instillation in his life that would become what people now recognize in him as courage. I agree. It is the "saddling up" and just doing it attitude that Willard, myself, and many others have come to live by.

"Have the courage to live. Anyone can die."

~ Attributed to Native American Robert "Tree" Cody

Willard learned from his mother's example, and he not only survived but thrived. He became, in his words, a mega over-achiever, challenging himself in sports, lettering in football and wrestling. He started his first business at age 19.

Along the way, however, Willard began to drink; a way that was popular, and he perceived would be good for numbing his mind and the buried anger and shame he felt from being "disabled". By age 13, he was using drugs, and by age 20 he was facing a five-year jail sentence. At age 24, he hit rock bottom mentally, emotionally, spiritually, physically, and financially. He recalls that at age 26, he was sober and free, but also homeless and ignorant. With 20 bucks to his name, he was clueless and unaware of the Laws of the Universe and how Life really works. At least he recognized and had the courage to acknowledge that all of his woes were self-induced.

What was also self-induced was the system he then developed and used to pull himself up from his despair. Quite unaware of what he was doing, *The Anatomy of Transformation* had begun. Through his own unconscious competence, he created his own system that not only turned all of those negative things around in his personal life, but that he also used unconsciously with his clients in his business consulting and coaching.

When I first heard Willard speak several years ago, I was impressed with his strength and sense of identity. His history of alcohol and drug abuse were simply facts of his past life. He lives sober, but doesn't think about it. Sobriety is just part of his new identity that he chose to create. He doesn't even *think* about having a drink. Recently, he put it this way, in his own words:

"I never liked the taste of alcohol; I drank it because I wanted to shut my mind off and affect my mood. I don't want to do that, now. That's not the being, the person that I am, so why would I ingest something I didn't like the taste of, and that the only reason I took it (in the first place) was to alter my mind? It's just not my identity anymore."

I know a thing or two about the wretched life of an alcohol and substance abuser. Our son Eric put himself and our family through 18 years of hell on earth, with his alcohol and drug abuse. There were countless times when we thought we'd lose him to an overdose, or one of the many suicide attempts, the crimes, the violence, drug dealings, arrests, and disappearances. He would go for periods of time, months, even years, estranged from the family. He was in and out of rehabs, and in and out of our lives, but never out of our hearts and thoughts. We lived in a constant state of exhausting anxiety, doing our best to work through our own emotions while looking for a successful resolution for him.

Listening to Willard speak gave me hope. At that time, Eric was sober again, and was rebuilding his life, but he was still estranged from our family. Fear, anger, and mistrust had come between us all, and the bitter past had left a deep scar on our hearts. Willard's teaching lifted my spirit. I saw a future for Eric, and for our family. I could choose to let go of the past, and love him unconditionally again! Love would be the catalyst that brought our family together again. Tears ran down my face as I released my anger and resentment. Once again, love for our son flooded my being. I imagined Eric meeting Willard. Eric would like him; they shared a zest for life. They would talk. Willard would encourage him, as he does so many others.

I resolved to get our son back. I was holding a ticket to a Tony Robbins event, and I would offer it to Eric. I envisioned Eric's awakening, and the beginning of the deep healing his soul craved. I knew the heart of this highly energetic being that I gave birth to. I knew his charismatic strengths, his leadership abilities, and his potential. I dreamed of his successful future and the unity of our family's nucleus, filled with laughter, love, and happy chaos.

Within a few months, Eric and I were reunited through texting. We reestablished trust and reconnected through love.

Daily fortifying his own courage, Eric was his lovable self again. He was excited about my ticket offer, and eagerly looked forward to attending the event. He never got that chance. He never got to meet Willard. I still have his ticket.

After Eric's death had rocked our entire Bazzy clan, one of my nephews, Joshua Bazzy Ph.D., a professor of psychology, approached me at a family gathering. Josh had an 'aha' moment as we spoke.

"Aunt Rachel, I never thought of how much courage it took Eric to keep starting over, again, and again."

A beautiful and profound observation that I appreciate and have always remembered.

Yes, it does take tremendous courage to pick yourself up, whether you are recovering from substance abuse, or starting over after a bankruptcy, or recovering from a failed relationship. It is courage that we call upon to pull ourselves up, and start over, and over, and over again. Willard's mother had the wisdom and courage to seek support and counsel for herself during his rock bottom years.

When it comes to Willard and his courage, he humbly doesn't perceive himself as a "courageous person", because he has observed that many people have a definition of what courage is to them; some people seem to think that courage is a suit of armor that they need to put on. We both agree that when the occasion arises, we just have to saddle up and face the situation, head on. The courage will develop along the way.

> "*Courage is not some thing that you do;*
> *it's a way of being, which brings the courage.*"
>
> ~ Willard Barth

No matter what any of us goes through, the BIG stuff is traumatic, and it feels like hell on earth to us. To someone else, perhaps it may not be that big of a deal. What is big and traumatic for one person is different for someone else. We shouldn't compare our experiences to someone else's as a way to measure (as if you could) "how much" courage each person has or lacks. Rather, each of us should reflect on our own experiences and circumstances, and measure courage by our own lessons and growth.

"Do or do not, there is no try."

~Yoda, Star Wars

Willard resists labeling himself as courageous, because to him, he's just done what he has had to do. Whether it was overcoming cancer, overcoming the drug use, overcoming the jail time, or overcoming being homeless, all these different things were met head on, with a "saddle up" attitude. He doesn't consider these "must do" scenarios as courageous acts. He is more prone to reserve the courage label for first responders and our military personnel. I concur; these special people are heroes, with a whole different level of courage unto their own.

I say, when you push yourself through difficult times, when you chose to "saddle up" and do what you need to do, the reward is your personal growth; you are strengthened, and your courage is increased. You learn valuable lessons, and remove another layer of self-doubt. You are reinventing yourself, every time you face a challenge head on.

I lay in darkness on the night Eric was killed, consumed with grief and exhausted; my insides felt like gelatin. In shock, and in what felt like a dark nightmare I wished I could wake up from, I was at the depths of the worst sorrow of my entire life. Somehow, from somewhere even deeper within me, rose the one, sane thought I recognized. It was the affirmation I learned from Tony Robbins. I grasped onto that thought, like a drowning woman would grasp a lifeline. Submerged in my despair, I pulled myself up from the depths, sobbing out the words, "Now, I am the voice. Now, I AM the voice. NOW, I AM THE VOICE". I repeated the entire affirmation through tears, over and over again, until I felt sane and grounded once more. There was an assurance within me from all of my studies and practices, all of my personal growth, and from my trust in my own wisdom. That was the night I learned to call on courage, like never before. That was the moment I chose to redirect my energy from focusing on my pain, to focusing on gratitude.

I fortified myself with a courage I didn't know was in me. I looked for anything and everything I could find to be grateful for. Yes, I cried. I cried a LOT. But I pushed myself to do what I needed to do. My family needed me. I needed me. I saddled up, broken hearted and all, and pushed myself, one step at a time, one day at a time.

And, if I can get through THAT, I can teach you how to do the same, no matter what you are facing in your life.

Go to willardbarthenterprises.com for more information on his transitional work

SIX

THE COURAGE TO LET GO

As I was creating the concept for this book, I got an idea to solicit several people of courage for their own, personal story that I could share with my readers. The objective is to offer you a broader spectrum of the many colors that courage shines through. As I proposed this concept to my elite circle of friends and colleagues, I was overwhelmed with offers from many of them, happy to share their "most courageous moment" with me for the benefit of all of us.

My beautiful friend and personal mentor, Peggy McColl, was one of the first people I interviewed, via a live, face to face call on our laptops. Peggy, being the professional that she is, had her perky story all ready for me, including the title,

"The Courage of Getting a Divorce".

We laughed together warmly.

Peggy McColl has been my mentor for over two years. She has usually been on the mentoring side of the lessons, conversations and emails, and more often than not, offering me assurance, advice, or being a good listener as I probed my way through the literary art and science of being a successful author. She is a *New York Times* Best Selling Author, an internationally recognized Speaker/Author/Mentor, and an expert in the area of goal achievement. I value her for so many reasons, however, what I admire about her most is her ability to create programs, write books, mentor souls like me, and promote prosperity in others, all while maintaining a total devotion to and the sustaining of her number one priority, which is her family.

Peggy, like myself and a lot of young girls growing up, dreamed of one day meeting the love of her life, getting married, having a family, and living happily ever after. Her dream partially came true in as much as she *did* meet a nice guy, and they *did* get married, and they *have* lived happily ever after, just not with each other! Not long into the marriage, they both realized it just wasn't going to work. They were from two different worlds, with different languages, values and priorities. There didn't seem to be a happy medium between them, and they were both mature enough to realize it was over. They resolved to becoming room-mates in a house they owned together, raising their son in neutral territory, sharing the mutual love they had for him.

As we spoke, Peggy recalled how much she was in love with her baby. I can relate, as most mothers can understand that feeling of a life growing within, and upon birth, seeing the What become a Who. Peggy relished in the unemployment she found herself in after the birth of their son, and enjoyed being a mid-thirty something, first time, stay-at-home mommy. She devoted all her time to loving and raising this perfect little person. In many ways (I deduced) her only child was and still is the love of her life.

As Peggy's intended story of *The Courage to Get a Divorce* unfolded, she laughed and recalled how she was eventually back in the workforce, but procrastinated moving out of their house on her own until her son was around two and a half years old. By then, she was a little more comfortable with him staying with other people while she was at work. We agreed that leaving your child in the custody of someone else does take courage, and faith, and it hurts like hell. Her story was, so far, so good, but I wanted more.

As Peggy ambled through her well thought out tale, she conceded that the time had come for her and her estranged husband to divorce. I am certainly inclined to believe that moving from a zone of comfort and familiarity out into the unknown, and being a single parent to boot, must have surely taken courage. I envisioned petite Peggy negotiating her way alone, baby in tow, through the perils of parenting, the housing market, a job, the bills, the decisions, and the gravity of having the sole responsibility for everything!

It takes a tremendous amount of courage to be on your own. I applaud the man or woman who has taken the necessary steps to raise their child in a safe environment of single parenting, despite the many challenges, compromises, and uncertainties. But, there is also a certain freedom in that "alone" period of one's life. Freedom to grow, to make decisions, and to examine core beliefs about oneself. There are opportunities to focus on truths, values, and gain a love and acceptance of who you are as a person. There is breathing room, as one heals from past wounds, and surges forward into Life once more.

As time passed, Peggy developed her skill sets as a parent, gained knowledge and wisdom in her professional life, and soared in her ability to "make things happen". She discovered her destiny as a mom, an author, an entrepreneur, and later as a mentor. She focused on what was important: her son and herself. To her credit, she has done a phenomenal job of it all, which is one of the many reasons I admire her.

As we conversed, swapping heartfelt thoughts about motherhood, Peggy mentioned that when her son went off to college, it nearly broke her heart! She missed him so terribly. I understood her emotions and the empty nest feelings that come when a kid moves out, even if they *do* return once in a while, with dirty laundry in hand. My husband and I have raised three children. I get it. As moms though, we love them so much, we want to decorate their apartments, buy them matching duvet and sheet sets, and make sure they have clean towels. It's our nesting instincts that drive us to be sure that all of their homey needs are met. *They* mostly want us to go away, so they can hang with their homies.

I'll always remember the time our two sons who, in their early 20s at the time, had to be practically pushed out of the nest! Our daughter who is the oldest, had already flown the coop; I had recovered sufficiently enough from missing her to realize that the next two needed their own place as well. It *was* rather sad, though, seeing my "baby" move on, but he needed to spread his wings and learn to be on his own, along with his street-wise older brother.

I would have never suspected that a year living with his older brother would turn into such a nightmare for our youngest, Zach. I worried about him constantly. Our older son began using drugs again and without us around to referee, the living situation for Zach became dreadful. Although I missed all three of our kids when they moved out, I did not miss the chaos that a drug addict brings to the family. It broke my heart, knowing that Eric was using again and that Zach was catching the brunt of Eric's behavior. I just wanted to protect them both a little longer, but I couldn't. They were young men, free to make their own decisions. It takes courage and faith to stand silently and watch your children grow up. I was greatly relieved for Zach's sake when their year's lease was up and they each went their own way.

I know how devoted Peggy is to her family. She adores her husband and dotes on her son, his wife, and now *their* son, her first grandchild. But when she recently began looking for a new home to move into, to be closer to her son and his family, he was the one who suddenly appeared to be the parent with the unwavering courage. He asked her to lunch, where he gently but firmly suggested she move on with her life, and not closer to his.

OUCH.

At least, that is what I was thinking. In Peggy's case, she thought about it too, spending a couple of days in tears, full of introspect and sorrow for the baby bird who was gone from the nest for good. She knew he was right, and that he absolutely meant her no harm, but she still ingested the suggestion and made herself nearly sick with grief by her perceived rejection. I looked at her through the camera of our connection and smiled at her with understanding. I've had three little chicka-dees move out into the world on their own. The first one was the hardest, our beautiful daughter, Leah; I can only imagine that when that first one is your *only* one, it can seem devastating.

Peggy, smiling a bit sheepishly, declared that she was in the process of mentally cutting the umbilical cord, and moving forward, as her son advised. She laughed as she ran her hand through her blond hair, adjusted her wire-framed glasses, and straightened her back, courageous and resilient.

"I guess he's more of a parent to me now than I am to him!" she chuckled.

"And THAT, my friend, is the name of your story", I replied. "*The Courage to Let Go*".

Ahhhhhhhhhh…

We as parents have to have the courage to let go, so they can fly. We have to release them as the children we remember in our minds, so they can become the adults that we can watch soar. We have to allow them to grow, make their own decisions, make their own mistakes, raise their families as they see fit, and have a life that doesn't necessarily center around our desires for them. We send them love, we stay close as a family, but not in proximity of every daily nuance and decision. We have to trust that we raised beautiful human beings who will be just fine and who will love us even more as time goes on, because they know we are always here for them if they need us.

And if we are very fortunate, we share our life with our children and even their children. We find our soulmate and our destiny of happily ever after is more than a girlish dream. I am one of these fortunate people and so is Peggy. By shifting her way of thinking, eventually Peggy manifested her dreamy husband. Practically love at first sight, Peggy's new neighbor Denis and she began a relationship that has grown into a beautiful marriage. Today, they are living in an abundance of love, joy, and prosperity. Peggy has also shifted her paradigm and now enjoys a healthier relationship with her son and his family and his freedom to soar on his own.

As for my husband and I, we are grateful that Eric never gave up on himself; we certainly didn't. But we *did* have to allow him to work it out himself. There were so many times when we thought we'd lose him to an overdose or suicide. There were countless incidents of crime, violence, anger, arrests, restitutions, disappearances, rehabs and second chances during the 18 years of hell he put our family and himself through when he was using. But, somewhere deep inside himself, he found the courage to pick himself up again and again. His resilience was a testimony to his inner strength. My husband and I each had the courage to continue to love him unconditionally.

> *"Eric, Mom loves you and*
> *I am never giving up on you."*
>
> ~ Rachel Bazzy, daily affirmation

Love wins. At the end of his short 32 years of life, Eric was living sober, he was happily married, had a good job, a nice home, his truck, and his motorcycle. We had reconciled our relationship with him and our lives were full of love, hope, and gratefulness. The night he was killed on his motorcycle forever changed the dynamic of our family. Heartbroken, I found a depth of courage to let go as I began the healing process. Just because I have moved on does not mean I have forgotten our son; I just have a destiny to fulfill. Eric will always be in my heart.

> *"God grant me the serenity to*
> *Accept the things I cannot change;*
> *Courage to change the things I can;*
> *And Wisdom to know the difference."*
>
> ~ Reinhold Niebuhr (1892-1971)

Is there someone or something in your life, a memory perhaps, a wound, or something or someone that you obsess over that you need to let go of? Every time you recall any of this negative "stuff", you are putting yourself in that negative vibration. Habitual thinking patterns that cause intense feelings of fear, anger, shame, or guilt are not only toxic, but also addictive in nature and become self-perpetuating. Carving neuropaths in the brain and creating a "super-highway" for thoughts to automatically race down, the thoughts automatically travel down the same road, coding it in deeper and deeper.

In order to change those pathways of toxic thoughts, those paradigms of negative thinking, we must first have the desire to change and then the *committed decision* to change. The value of that decision depends upon the courage that is required to make the choice and stick to the commitment. In other words, it takes courage to let go. The good news is, if you will commit today to letting go of just one negative thought or idea, and replace it with its opposite, positive thought, and continually focus on that positive idea, you *will* see the change over time.

By purposely guarding your thoughts and interrupting the old story running through your mind (again), you will form the habit of thinking more and more in a positive light. Peggy and I have both mastered the courage it takes to be the moms we are today. The following quote by Portia Nelson uniquely illustrates the thinking patterns of human beings and how to change them.

I

I walk down the street.
There is a deep hole in the sidewalk.
I fall in.
I am lost...
I am hopeless.
It isn't my fault.
It takes forever to find a way out.

II

I walk down the same street.
There is a deep hole in the sidewalk.
I pretend I don't see it.
I fall in again.
I can't believe I'm in the same place.
But it isn't my fault.
It still takes a long time to get out.

III

I walk down the same street.
There is a deep hole in the sidewalk.
I see it is there.
I still fall in...it's a habit.
My eyes are open; I know where I am;
It is my fault.
I get out immediately.

IV

I walk down the same street.
There is a deep hole in the sidewalk.
I walk around it.

V

I walk down another street.

~ Portia Nelson, American singer, song writer, actress, author
(5/27/1920 – 3/6/2001)

Thinking of writing a book? Go to peggymccoll.com for more information

SEVEN

COURAGE IS A VERB

I have a huge heart for immigrants; people coming to America, looking for a better way of life. I get it. I see their hunger, their desperation, their desire for a chance to just feed their families and make a decent living. People from around the world look to our United States' shores to escape poverty, violence, persecution, and political conflict in their own homeland. For so many, hope is a four letter word. They are beyond hope; they are desperate.

"Give me your tired, your poor, your huddled masses
Yearning to breathe free"

~ Emma Lazarus,
Sonnet on the base of the Statue of Liberty

I believe that too many people give little more than a passing thought to those who strive to come to America today, yearning for a better life. It's as if the phrase "Give me your poor" is just an old colloquialism from a bygone era of our ancestors, you know, from back in the late 1700s. But, let's face it; unless you were born as a Native American Indian, we are *all* descendants from a courageous forefather who faced unfathomable odds in seeking freedom, liberty, and an opportunity for a more desirable life.

My husband's grandfather immigrated to America, according to census records, from Syria in 1914. With nothing but the clothes on his back and a few coins in his pocket, he sought a better life. He didn't speak any English. When he was processed on Ellis Island in Upper New York Bay, the U.S. Bureau of Immigration didn't know how to spell his last name, Bazzi, so it was recorded as Bazzy. That's how the Bazzy family got here. That's only two generations ago from our era.

My father-in-law, who is now 88, has shared with us many a tale of his father's struggles upon arrival to America; the poverty, the lack, and the hard, physical labor of grinding out a meager existence in an Eastern European immigrant neighborhood of Detroit, Michigan. Chris' dad was pulled from school and put to work as a young boy, running one of his father's butcher shops, while Mr. Bazzi oversaw the second location he'd scraped together with a relative. Their family lived as tenants upstairs, over the shop, and existed off the meat that was too brown to sell, and leftover, overly-ripened fruits and vegetables from the shop down below. Dad translated the Arabic his father spoke into English for the customers, suppliers, and vendors; he kept the books straight, ran the errands, and delivered crates twice his weight.

I can trace *my* ancestry, on the other hand, back over five generations of proud Texans; all the way back to when the Texas territory was the Republic of Texas in 1836 and beyond. My 1800s kinsmen were white-bread, home-fed, Bible thumping farmers, scratching out a living off the land, and courageously fighting for religious, political, and civil freedoms. Some were German immigrants. My Proud Texan roots go deep. Seeing the Alamo in my hometown of San Antonio, where some of my ancestors lost their lives in battle for freedom, still chokes me up.

I have many courageous friends who have immigrated to America, but one of those who most exemplifies courage in my mind is our dear friend, Andi Duli, because he never gave up. Andi has got to be one of the most courageous, *persistent* people I know and that is one of the main things that it takes to see your dreams come true. Andi is now somewhat of a folk hero in the network marketing circles; he shares his story of courage and determination from the stage in order to encourage others to pursue their dreams. I recently had the opportunity to sit down with Andi while we were attending a national convention together and we talked about many things, including the defining, courageous moments in his life.

"Everything can be taken from a man but one thing:
the last of the human freedoms – to choose one's attitude in
any given set of circumstances, to choose one's own way."

~ Dr. Viktor E. Frankl
Neurologist, Psychiatrist, Holocaust survivor

Andi was born and raised in Albania, when it was still a communist state. For the first 18 years of his life, he lived in a government controlled environment of lack; lack of food, lack of utilities, lack of opportunities, and lack of hope. His family's home had electricity for two hours in the morning and two hours in the evening. They had limited running water; again, two hours in the morning and a couple of hours in the evening. Food was scarce; citizens were issued coupons for milk and bread, and stood in long lines for hours and hours, many times having to return to their homes empty-handed. Most nights, Andi and his family went to bed hungry.

Many of us in this country of the United States of America can hardly relate to such abject scarcity, unless you have experienced living in an area after a natural disaster has occurred, when there is no clean water or food. Even then, thankfully, the help comes pouring in from neighboring cities, states, and government programs. I dare say that the average panhandler on the street eats better than Andi and his family did back then under that Marxist-Leninist regime in Albania.

I was further dismayed as I listened to Andi describe the day when he went to stand in line for milk at 5 o'clock in the morning. Little ten-year old Andi walked alone in the cold, pre-dawn hours to relieve his father who had already been standing in line for *three hours* for a meager, government ration of milk. His father left to go to work while Andi continued to wait patiently in line for several more hours, along with all of the other desperate people. He recalled that he was the third person from the front of the line when the cashier suddenly announced that there was no more milk. His spirit sank. People left, disheartened. Ten-year old Andi stood there shivering with emotion, unwilling to give up. Tears rolled down his innocent face as he remained behind, lamenting to the cashier, in between his sobs, that there had to be one more bottle of milk! His baby sister needed the milk! His pleading fell on deaf ears; the milk truck was long gone. I can just imagine this sweet little boy, as he cried with anguish, making his way back home, his efforts futile. It was a defining moment in his young life.

That was just under 30 years ago, folks! This isn't some anecdotal story from the horse and buggy days of the 1800s. This is *in our lifetime*. Andi is just a few years older than our daughter! I wouldn't want my child to endure that life! Andi's folks weren't a couple of uneducated, dumb-lucks; his father was an engineer and the head of his company, and his mother was the principal of a school. Yet together, in this regulated environment, they barely made $520 of combined salaries a month. Yet, it wasn't for lack of money that they starved; it was because of the circumstances of a culture of communist autarky, desperate economics, and government refusal to trade with the outside world.

Citizens in Albania had no voice; there was absolutely NO complaining allowed, under threat of the *death penalty* for conspiring against the state. The citizens were basically hostages, isolated from the outside world. NO one was allowed to leave. Their news media was limited and controlled; there was only one local T.V. station. Anyone caught with an antenna for receiving outside channels was prosecuted and killed. A penal code required the death penalty for anyone over the age of 11, who was found guilty for conspiring against the state, damaging state property, or committing economic sabotage. The definition of each of those charges was open for interpretation by the state. There were no civil rights. Political executions were common, with an estimated 25,000 people who were killed under this time period of communist regime in Albania. Looking back, Andi still refers to it as "living the Albanian nightmare".

Listening as Andi spoke, and hearing of the abject poverty and desperation he was raised in back then, caused an empathic shake of my head in sympathy and wonder. I am humbled by the unmeasurable courage it must have taken to survive in such a destitute environment. This was no circus. There were no parties, festive meals, bountiful holidays, or paid vacations. Andi had never tasted candy or chocolate, licked the icing off a cupcake, or accidentally spilled his milk. *There was no milk to spill!*

This Marxist rule controlled everything. Declaring themselves an atheist state, the communist authorities launched a violent campaign to extinguish all religious life in Albania, forcing the closing of all churches, mosques, monasteries, and other religious institutions. They abolished all European and any other foreign influences.

Can you even imagine existing in a country that has no freedom of speech or press?! A place where there is no freedom of expression in the arts, theater, literature, dance, or in music? Imagine being trapped in a political culture that prohibits religious freedom and has no foundation of faith, no spirituality, no moral code. No cause for hope. Can you imagine living in an environment that doesn't encourage any virtues like courage, or gratitude, or the Golden Rule; that doesn't allow the study of personal growth, or the striving for success? Even after the eventual, total collapse of communism in Albania, the new Democratic Party made empty promises, and caused further desperate and economic corruption.

Growing up, Andi heard a few, whispered stories of a cousin who somehow escaped Albania to begin a new life in Italy or another who made it out and started a business in Greece. They were successful – they were free. These rare stories fed Andi's burning desire. Growing up, he would imagine that he also would also leave Albania someday, somehow, some way. He constantly held this dream, this idea of freedom in his mind. He felt, knew, that he would get out of Albania and to a better life. His vision was to have a free life and to be able to help his parents financially.

For most of his youth, Andi spoke these statements of freedom out loud to himself, to his family, and his closest friends. The more he spoke it out loud, the more he believed it; and the more he believed it, the more inspired he became. He harbored a burning desire and a crystal clear picture in his mind, never allowing his outside environment to dissuade him from his dream. Finally, one day the dream started becoming a reality.

> *"The greatest discovery was the power of*
> *the subconscious mind touched by faith.*
> *In every human being is that limitless reservoir*
> *of power which can overcome*
> *any problem in the world."*

~ William James, Father of American Psychology

When Andi turned age 18, he begged his father to help him get to the United States to attend college. The Albanian borders were open under the new Democratic Party; however, only a very limited number of applicants per day would be accepted for a Visa. Andi applied for his Visa and was not accepted. He applied again, believing that acceptance was supposed to happen, that he was supposed to receive his salvation. As if by divine decree, he was one of three people one day who were granted a Visa. Now, he stood determined presenting his case to his parents.

> *"Dad, please help me get to America!*
> *If you help me get there,*
> *if you give me a chance, I WILL pay you back.*
> *I WILL help the family. I WILL help support you guys."*

There's an old, documented saying that has been circulating since the early 1800s, "Where there's a will, there's a way". Actually, there is a lot of universal truth in that statement. The Will is one of our six higher mental faculties. As Bob Proctor teaches, the only limitation we have is weakness of attention and poverty of imagination.

Through our creative imagination we can "see" ourselves where we want to be using our mental eyes and feel ourselves in that state of being. When we are courageous enough to allow ourselves to use our imagination to dream, when we get emotionally charged with our goal, we impress this into our subconscious mind. By persistently visualizing our goal as accomplished and holding that thought in our mind, seeing our outcome as happening *now* in present tense, then we are operating within the Laws of the Universe.

Our Will is what is used to *focus* our attention on a specific goal. Our Will gives us the ability to use the energy and power that is flowing through our consciousness, and concentrate it on a specific idea, thought, or picture in our mind. We hold that thought and keep it alive and burning with desire by using our Will. It takes courage to allow yourself to do this. That is why a developed courage is so very important.

Ralph Waldo Emerson, one of America's foremost transcendental philosophers, stated, "A man is what he thinks about all day long". Dr. Joseph Murphy, in his book, *The Power of Your Subconscious Mind*, teaches us, "When you begin to control your thought processes, you can apply the powers of your subconscious to any problem or difficulty." Unwittingly, Andi had spent his youth training his mind, and reprogramming his subconscious with his belief in his freedom and his success in America. Now this young man was putting his courage into action.

"To believe is to accept something as true, or to live in the state of being it; as you sustain this mood, you shall experience the joy of the answered prayer!"

~ Dr. Joseph Murphy
Psychologist, Author

As Andi's father considered the opportunity that his son presented to him, his mother worried about her only son.

Eventually, Andi convinced both of them with his optimism and his burning desire. His father proposed a venture with his company, parlayed company stock, and invested everything he had into his son's future.

Next, Andi had to approach the principal of his school for permission to withdraw from school early. His courage was fueled by his desire to help his family. His faith was increased by his successful Immigrant Visa process. Now he was believing in the impossible: early discharge from school, when he hadn't finished the year's courses. And, his grade point average, well, frankly it sucked.

"I don't care what somebody has in their head.
It's what's in their heart".

~ Andi Duli

When I asked Andi about having the courage to plead with his dad to put the milk money on the line, and to petition the school principal to grant him clearance, Andi replied,

"I asked. Sometimes we've got to ask for the impossible."

Andi had made a pledge that he would find a way to help financially support his parents and siblings. He held the dream of a better life in his mind. He reinforced his desire with positive thoughts, speech, and affirmations. He believed so strongly in the unseen and had faith in an unexplainable *knowing* in his gut. He literally *spoke* the positive into his life.

Finally, with all of his documents and papers in order, Andi and his family took an emotional ride to the airport. Andi continued to reassure his parents that he was on his chosen path; that he was drawn to this, it was his calling. He was going to be free, and he was going to help support them. He committed to never looking back. There were a lot of tears, as they spent these last moments together. Andi remained strong and optimistic. Life would never be the same.

Andi hugged and kissed his family good-bye, then went through the gate, never looking back. Afterwards, as he sat alone on a jet he had never experienced, he shed his tears of departure, and of new beginnings. He knew no English, had only a small suitcase of clothing, and a few hundred dollars to his name, but finally, *he was free!*

The long flight finally landed in Atlanta, Georgia – an airport that seemed bigger than his small hometown! He went to the nearest burger joint, hungry and thirsty, not able to speak any English, and unable to communicate his order. The woman behind the counter couldn't understand him, so she blew him off in her rush to help the next person in line. Embarrassed over his ignorance of the English language, Andi left the establishment thinking, "What's another day of going hungry and thirsty?"

Living in a dormitory on campus, Andi immersed himself in trying to learn English, but it was very difficult. Within a few months, summer arrived and the dorms closed for the season. Andi got a small apartment to rent and slept on the floor because he couldn't afford furniture. He delivered pizza on a bicycle that a friend gave him. Andi had heard that in order to become free in this country, you go to school for four years, get a degree, put in 40 years' worth of work, make 40 thousand a year, which to him was a *fortune*, and then you retire. He had taken action, got himself to America, did what he had heard, and went to college. His struggles were antagonizing.

After many years of frustration and failure, Andi was no closer to his goal of graduating from college. Now in his mid-20s, having married his girlfriend while they were in college, he struggled to support himself and his loving wife. More years passed until one day it dawned on him, "HEY, I didn't come to America to be a pizza delivery guy!"

Andi was at a very low point in his life. Now he was working two jobs delivering pizza and working in an ice cream store. His dreams were slipping further and further away. He had applied for so many jobs, filled out countless applications, and struggled for so long to keep his hopes alive. Andi felt dejected. He was desperate. He perceived that no one gave him a chance; he had no experience, no degree, and no connections. He had just wanted an opportunity; he felt rejected, tired, and was struggling. Working long, hard hours, he drove a beat-up old car that a friend gave him, which had the embarrassing mechanical flaw of insistent honking, almost as if the car had its own free will. Andi's faith was dwindling along with his immense disappointment.

By age 30, Andi was at rock bottom financially. He was broke, $40,000 in debt, credit cards maxed out, and about to lose his home and his marriage. Focusing on everything that was wrong with his life, Andi was deeply in pain over his entire situation. He beat himself up for his immaturity, for his lack of skills, and his poor English. He held resentments in his heart against people he felt had hurt him or screwed him somehow. Andi held unforgiveness towards people, and I dare say, towards himself as well. Although free, he was not living his American dream and he felt miserable and defeated.

One day, his wife suggested that he take out a pen and paper and write down everything he was feeling; all of the hurts, the resentments, the disappointments, the negativity... all of it, and then burn it. Andi listened. Andi took action. He wrote out page after page, filled with his mental anguish; he then burned it as a symbolic way of releasing it all. He says that as the smoke wafted away, he could feel the burden lift off his shoulders. The ashes of his renewed faith made fertile ground for the seeds of hope that were about to be planted. It was another defining moment in his life; the courage to face his truths and change his attitude. His heart was now open for opportunity once more.

Soon after, still looking for a better job, Andi was invited to attend a direct selling marketing event. He ran into an old friend whom Andi knew had lost everything, his cars, his house, his finances, and now here he stood, dressed in a fine, expensive suit, and wearing custom, alligator shoes! Surprised, Andi asked his buddy what had happened! What changed? His friend replied that he had *remembered to dream again*. He took action. He made changes in his attitude, and now he was back in prosperity. Andi recalls the challenge:

> "*If you can dream one more time,*
> *get excited one more time…*"

This supportive friend exposed Andi to high level thinking. He gave him a DVD about network marketing and planted the seeds of success in his fertile mind. Andi now had a 30,000 foot view of his situation and his hope was renewed. Inspired, Andi retrained himself to believe in the dream of success again, renewed his forgotten habits of positive thinking, and recommitted himself to his goals. With regards to that turning point in his life, Andi shared this with me:

> "*When you go through the valley, it's a scary thing to dream,*
> *but dreaming is the only way people get out of their situation.*"

> ~ Andi Duli

I agree. It takes renewed courage to dream again, to see beyond where you are, and to visualize where you want to be. I challenge you to have the courage to let go of the past; your past does not define you. It's not what has happened to you; it's about what you do about what happened to you. You can choose to hold on to the past, the hurts, the pains, the self-pity, and all of the other negative thoughts, and live a miserable, hum-drum existence, OR you can let it go.

"When anything happens:

1. It is what it is. Accept it. You cannot change it.
It will either control you, or you will control it.

2. Harvest the Good.
The more you look for it, the more you'll find.

3. Forgive all of the rest.
Forgive means to let go of completely, abandon."

~ Michael Bernard Beckwith
New Thought Minister, Author, Founder

Make a committed decision today. Your attitude is your choice. Developing your Courage is your choice. Nothing and no one can take away your freedom to choose your own thoughts.

Today, Andi Duli is enjoying his boyhood dreams of living in freedom, prosperity, and being able to financially help out his family back in Albania. Once he used courage to dream again, his life began to turn around. He heart was open to new ideas, new opportunities, and better relationships. Andi continues to study personal growth, is always looking to improve himself, and is a tremendous encouragement to everyone with whom he comes in contact. His imperfect English is part of his charm. His great heart is what makes him successful.

Andi and his precious wife are blissfully married. They travel the world together, live in their beautiful dream home, and enjoy and share their prosperity and success. Together they have built a dream team of over 15,000 people with annual sales of over $30 million and growing. Andi hasn't needed perfect grammar to take action, to persevere, and to go after his dreams.

It takes courage to pull yourself up, renew your faith, and believe in your dream, *just one more time.* As you strengthen your courage muscle, you will find that the bounce-back gets easier and easier. The true goal is to sustain that optimal attitude of persistence, trust in the Laws of the Universe, and have gratitude for the journey you are on. Today is a new day, no matter where the sun is shining. Be Courageous. You'll thank yourself later for what you do for yourself today.

"Think strongly,
Attempt fearlessly,
Accomplish masterfully."

~ James Allen,
British Philosophical Writer

EIGHT

BAD COMPANY

While contemplating the contents for this chapter, I asked Spirit for guidance. That guidance came as I slept, reminding me of an event in my childhood. The recollection of that day shows me vividly the events that occurred, although I haven't thought about it in years. It was when I was a very young child, perhaps around four years old. I was at my grandmother's house one day, playing with my older cousins. Their mom and my mom went shopping together with our grandmother, leaving us in the care of another adult.

We were outside playing as usual, when my cousins began picking innocently flowers from the next-door neighbor's flowerbeds on the side of the house. I recall that they encouraged me to join them, so I did. We then proudly took our gift inside my grandparent's home to present to our babysitter. She was *not* pleased. I was confused.

Examining the evidence, she proceeded to interrogate the perpetrators of this appalling crime of stealing. I was still confused, as I stood in the living room with the pretty flowers now seemingly burning in my little hands. *Stealing?* I had no concept of what stealing really meant except that, "Thou shalt not steal" was taught in Sunday School. She proceeded to lecture us on taking what wasn't ours, and yes, that included the flowers from someone else's yard. She sent us all out of the room, then brought us each back in, one at a time, to further accuse, sentence, and punish with a good beating on the backside. I don't recall the order, but I *do* remember the dread of waiting for my turn, while listening to the commotion and wailing in the next room.

We were then marched out the front door, down the steps, and over to the neighbor's front door, so we could give her the flowers from her garden and apologize for stealing them. The neighbor was surprisingly sweet, forgave us, and dismissed the crime with kindness. She accepted the flowers and our tearful confessions, granting us absolution. We were then marched home, separated, and told to "go think about what you've done". All I could think was that it wasn't fair! A terrible injustice had been done, in my four-year-old mind. I was innocent! They made me do it. They, being older, should have known better. I didn't know that I was stealing!

I've long since forgiven our babysitter for her harsh punishment that day, and my cousins for their part in the fiasco. It wasn't funny back then, but as I write about it now, it makes me chuckle. Perhaps that event happened for me, so I could learn not to unjustly serve as a judge and jury for others.

"Shoot first, ask questions later"

Apparently shooting first, metaphorically speaking, and asking questions later, ran in the family. Another incident when I was around four years old occurred. My younger brother was a baby at the crawling stage. As my mother was putting him down for a nap one afternoon, I noticed that the toilet paper was completely unrolled all over the floor of our small bathroom. I figured my baby brother had discovered it and had gotten curious. I didn't want him to get a spanking, so I knelt down and began quickly rolling it back on the cardboard tube. I was startled when my mother came around the corner and "caught me". I was even more surprised when she jerked me up from the floor and spanked me good and hard.

I remember her sternly chastising me as my chest heaved with shock and tears. I should know better. Why did I do that? Between sobs, I finally could explain that I *didn't* do it, *Danny Boy* did, and I didn't want him to get in trouble. Now it was *her* turn to cry. She held me in her arms as we sat in her rocking chair, both of us crying and her apologizing to me over and over. I can still see the regret and sadness in her face; parent fail 101. Bless her heart. I love you, Mother.

These may be endearing memories now; however, I am very aware that these and other events of accusation contributed to the paradigm in my developing childhood mind. Growing up in an environment of strict religious doctrine, I imagined that I needed to be as good as I could be so I wouldn't get into trouble or go to hell. I had to be a good example for others. There was no room for failure without immediate punishment. Failure was bad. Failure was a sin. By the time I was an adult, I was a full-blown people pleaser, serving others to the best of my abilities. I kept a perfect house, made sure my kids were always clean and well behaved. I volunteered at church, and served on the PTA. I was the gymnastics and soccer team mom, the car-pooler, the banner making, gym mural painting, enthusiastic cheerleader; then I went to work for my husband. That's an exhausting way to believe, trying to live a life perfectly in order to earn others love, including our Creator's love.

Up until just a few years ago, I lived with an unidentified paradigm that made me somehow think I wasn't good enough. I felt that I was in trouble when my name was called. I had an unknown guilt for an unknown reason. Similar to seeing a police car's lights in your rear-view mirror, I would start searching my mind for what was wrong. I'd feel guilty or accused, and start coming up with possible scenarios in my mind, creating the excuse, alibi, or reason for whatever it was that I imagined. Later on, the reasoning turned into a verbal "come-back" for any perceived attack through aggressive teasing. I had a sharp sense of humor so the return barb to the opponent was funny and all done in jest, but frankly, deep down, it was a defense for my own low esteem.

As I studied further in human psychology and self-awareness, I finally recognized this type of humor as harmful. I realized that I didn't want to live that way anymore. Adopting a stronger courage within, I stopped the bad habit cold turkey. I made a commitment that I would no longer engage in the sarcastic, passive-aggressive banter with those who communicated in this type of rapport.

"Sometimes it takes more courage to be quiet
than it does to speak up."

~ Rachel Bazzy

As I continued my studies, I began to realize my own worth. I stopped the nonsense in my head from the old paradigms and replaced it with positive thoughts and affirmations. Paying close attention to the language I used, both verbally and in my mind, I raised my own standard, and began treating everyone with love and respect, including myself. And by the way, the teasing barbs from others ceased and better relationships developed.

*"You are the by-product of other people's
habitual way of thinking."*

~ James Arthur Ray

Have you ever questioned where you got the ideas that you currently live with? I highly encourage you to take a few minutes, engage your courage, and examine your thoughts, verbiage, and ideals. What sort of rules are you living by? What limiting beliefs do you have? Are you happy, prosperous, confident, and successful? Or are you depressed, living in lack, fearful, and anxious? Are you suffering or soaring? Surviving or thriving? Are you positive and optimistic or do you have negative thoughts and are self-deprecating?

We are all born with a DNA code formed from our ancestors, which is why your kid has Grandpa's nose, and you put your shoes and socks on in a certain order. There is a genetic and environmental programing in all of us from the minute we are born. Everything we hear, see, feel, and experience is recorded in our subconscious mind. Our environment shapes our thinking when we are young, and unless we make a conscious decision to change a bad habit or negative thought and replace it with something better, we will be nothing more than just another brick in the wall, as the Pink Floyd song goes.

We are born with an inherited DNA; all the physical and spiritual attributes and dispositions, temperament, mannerisms, propensities, and thought processes, to name a few. Have you ever been told you're always late just like Aunt so-and-so, or do you never seem to have enough money just like your parents or grandparents? Do you think you have a bad temper because you're Irish? These attributes may be inherited as part of our DNA, but our relatives or friends who recognize and reinforce them are *programming* us to believe and live out those cues like a virus in our subconscious computer.

We are the accumulation of a genetic pool that dates back for many generations, *plus* the viral coding of our environment. We have a certain predisposition, an inclination or tendency as we grow up, *attracting more* of what we already are without the realization why. Unless we are taught how to become aware and alter this genetic coding in our subconscious, this paradigm will continue to give us what we've always had, and we will be what we've always been. This is more than physical characteristics. It is a virus that distorts our values, blinds us from what is really important, and twists the Universal Truths, robbing us of the fulfillment we could be enjoying in our lives.

In 2013 a study led by neuroscientists at Emory University found that genetic markers, previously thought to be wiped clean before birth, were used to transmit a single traumatic experience across generations. The researchers exposed male mice to the scent of cherry blossoms and associated that smell with a mild shock to the feet of the mice. Later, when bred with female mice that were not exposed to the trauma, the resulting pups were raised in a neutral environment until full grown. When the cherry blossom scent was introduced for the first time to this next offspring, the mice suddenly became anxious and fearful. This "memory transmission" also extended out to the next generation when these mice were bred.

Now that's a sketchy thought. We don't know exactly *what* we have inherited from our ancestors!

It's not our fault, but say it with me, *it is our problem*. We are good people, but the company we keep in our minds and DNA determines our outcomes in our lives. It is up to each one of us to examine, recognize, and break the epigenetic inheritance, eliminating the programing and the paradigms that we have lived under, and start living a more fulfilling, purpose driven life. *This takes courage.* Which brings me to the very intriguing story of my friend, Amber.

Royal Amber spent a portion of her childhood traveling the world with her parents, living in various countries, with assorted traditions and environments. Her folks returned to the United States from Italy when Amber was about four years old. By the time she was six, she was living the simple life with her family on one of the islands of Fiji. Amber's family lived in a small, modest home on the property; her father managed the resort on the isolated 4.7 square mile island while her mother tended to her own duties. More times than not, Amber chose to stay with the local village people more than her parents at the resort. She spent her childhood barefoot, with no cars, no Western clothes, and no electricity, trading modern conveniences for the feeling of unity and acceptance within the Fijian community.

A boat would arrive once a month with supplies. Island visitors were few and far in between. Amber learned from her Fijian family how to spear-fish for food, tend the garden, feed the chickens, cook their native dishes, and speak the language in this Third World country setting. She absorbed the customs, attended school, learned the traditional dances and songs, and lived a simple life that was rich in culture and history.

I have spent time in Fiji, and not only is it incredibly beautiful, the indigenous people are some of the most hospitable, friendly, soft-spoken souls I have ever encountered. I can imagine being a child growing up there, with the endless horizon of the South Seas, the scented rainforests, splashing waterfalls, pristine beaches, and black-velvet skies glittering with millions of stars at night. There were hills to climb and coral reefs full of exotic fish to explore. I can imagine a young Amber shimmying up a palm tree or racing with the other kids down a jungle forest path. Life was full of adventure, challenges, and village unity.

Amber recalls being the only young, white girl on the island, and the daughter of the manager of a millionaire's own Bali Hai. At age four, while previously living in the USA, she remembers having been sexually molested twice. She didn't understand what was happening and kept it to herself, too afraid to speak up about the occurrences. Now, on this remote island in the South Pacific, from the age of six through age eleven, she was again being violated by various, young courters who just wanted her attention. In retrospect, Amber justified for herself that they meant no real harm; each boy or teenager seemed to want to earn the favor of this fair-skinned, blond beauty so that someday when she left the island, she would take him with her. Amber was sexually molested nine times by nine different persons; it was courting that went too far, *especially* when it involved a child. Naive and confused, she told no one.

At age 12 Amber moved back to the States with her family, who settled in Los Angeles, California. Her parents worked all the time and Amber felt alone. She felt she had no one. After the adventurous life she had lived in Fiji, she sought and found a "village" of her own in the form of a gang. The gang did "exciting" things, which made her feel a part of something once again. Amber learned a new slang language and the ways of the violent culture to which she was now exposed. She had no idea what she was getting into; she was with bad company, and in way over her head. She was raped for the first time at age twelve.

Amber was raped again at age 14. This time, her parents were made aware of the sexual assault. Amber recalls that the perpetrator threatened the family with violence, saying he would kill them all if they reported the incident. Ultimately, out of fear, they agreed to do nothing, leaving Amber feeling rejected and insignificant.

One day Amber was hanging out at a drug dealer's house with one of her gang friends. The guy fixed up a drug for her and her friend. The 14 year old had never done drugs before, so she didn't listen to the instructions very closely. Instead of taking the "one hit", Amber took 20 to 30 hits and accidentally overdosed. Everything went black. She was out of her body. Terrified, Amber was looking down on the scene below, her body slumped back, mouth slack, and eyes fixed in a coma-like gaze. Hovering over her limp form, she heard, "No, it's not time for you to leave", and then everything went black once more. Fifteen minutes had passed when she finally came to and realized she was back in her body. She had somehow survived an overdose that would have killed an elephant. After that experience she stopped fearing death and the fear of wondering "do you go on afterwards?" Amber felt that now that she knew the answer, the fear of death was gone.

At 16 Amber met a nice guy from a different gang in L.A. and they began dating. This inter-dating between gangs was unacceptable, but he sheltered her from the other gang members; he saved her life and kept her away from the gang violence. He would "get her out" when things got too rough. She fell in love and they dated for several years. Meanwhile, she was still sneaking out of her parents' house and hanging with her homegirls in the old gang.

When she was 17, Amber found herself in trouble with the law, leaving her with a Class II felony on her record! She didn't give up, however. At the end of her first year of college, she joined the military. Eventually, her record was expunged, and Amber was accepted into the Armed Services. Stationed at a holding area, waiting for boot camp to begin, as unbelievable as it may seems, an unidentified guard *violently* raped her! She decided to just "let it go", using the experience to further drive her towards her goal of protecting others. At 21 she had developed the courage to push through, no matter what. She decided enough was enough and took control of her life.

"Stand in your power; remember who you are.
You came here with a gift – use it!"

~ Royal Amber Rojas

Undeterred, Amber stood in her strength, serving three years with the Military Police Company. She was an excellent marksman, earning citations, recognitions, and an Army Achievement medal. After her honorable discharge, Amber returned to finish college. She then applied for the Police Academy and eventually served the community on the police force for several years. Her courage and mental shift set her free of the generational curse of victimization.

Whether we are aware of repetitive behaviors and events or not, our subconscious *will* attract more of whatever is currently in our lives. I don't believe that a four-year-old child consciously attracts sexual molestation or victimization of any sort. Children don't develop cognition until they reach an age between five to seven years old. Cognitive skills are the skills the brain used to think, learn, remember, pay attention, and solve problems. A four year old has memory and imagination and sees things symbolically. Perhaps our epigenetic inheritance puts us in situations that facilitate events and experiences that then lead to further attraction to similar circumstances, repeating the outcomes until one day, we become aware and choose to change our programming.

*"It's not what happens to us; it's what
we do about what happens to us."*

~ Rachel Bazzy

As for Amber and myself, we are both dedicated to helping other people through sharing our stories, wisdom, and experiences. It takes a tremendous amount of courage and faith to get through sexual abuse and come out the other side stronger and more self-realized. Amber uses her experiences to fuel her determination to help others who have experienced trauma.

I think some people don't give themselves enough credit for the courage within. *Our Source for Courage is Infinite.* We can tap into that source through prayer, meditation, and/or focused desire. We have to have courage to develop ourselves to our fullest potential. I in-courage you to focus on who you want to be. Let the past go. TODAY is your day to awaken.

*"In the barque of your soul reclines the commanding Master;
he does but sleep; wake him.
Self-control is strength; Right Thought is mastery;
Calmness is power."*

~ James Allen, *As a Man Thinketh*

NINE

GLASS HOUSES

We walk this path of Life together, you and me. We are all connected, whether you realize it or not. It's okay if you aren't quite as aware of this as some people are, but it is not okay to remain in ignorance, once the subject of Oneness or personal growth has been brought to your attention. Living in an ignorant state keeps us in bondage. The key to freedom is knowledge, and knowledge comes from studying.

> *"We are all connected; To each other, biologically.*
> *To the earth, chemically.*
> *To the rest of the universe, atomically."*

~ Neil deGrasse Tyson, American Astrophysicist

If this seems like "New Age thought" to you, or feels contradictory to your current belief system, that's actually a good sign. It means it's time for you to explore the possibilities within your own mind, and stop being a sheeple (sheep-like people: docile, ignorant, or easily led). All of humanity should be on a journey of growth, learning, and improving. I humbly suggest you don't worry or criticize yourself or others, my friend, because we each have to start somewhere.

Begin where you are today. This book was divinely guided into your hands! Listen, if we aren't growing, we're dying. If we aren't moving forward, we're in reverse. *There is no sitting still in Life.* We are made up of particles of energy and energy is always moving. I invite you to have the courage to open your mind, consider thoughts that may be new to you, and contemplate your current belief system. There's nothing weird or unusual about this; it's quantum mechanics.

> *"I am saddened by how people treat one another*
> *and how we are so shut off from one another and*
> *how we judge one another, when the truth is,*
> *we are all one connected thing.*
> *We are all from the same exact molecules."*
>
> ~ Ellen DeGeneres

Many of us are familiar with the expression, "People who live in glass houses shouldn't throw stones". This is a centuries old proverb that started in European countries, which basically means that one should not criticize others, because everybody has faults of one sort or another. The Cambridge Dictionary supports the expression to mean that we should not criticize others for a poor quality in their character, which we most likely harbor in ourselves. Basically, it is a warning not to be hypocritical.

You know, there are way too many people in this world who are critical, judgmental, self-righteous, sarcastic, or just plain grumpy. It seems like there's an epidemic of judging one another. There is a constant media influx of complaining, criticism, attacks of character, and exploitation of human flaws; there's ridicule, condemnation, and disapproval, and snarkiness.

Suddenly, everyone's a critic! None of us are perfect – if we were, there would be no room for growth and expansion, and Spirit is always looking for growth and expansion.

"We can never judge the lives of others, because each person knows only their own pain and renunciation. It's one thing to feel that you are on the right path, but it's another to think yours is the only path."

~ Paulo Coelho

If you think you are passively watching, listening to, or agreeing with any of the brouhaha out there, you are just as guilty as those who are actively perpetuating this negative habit of gross "news and entertainment"; the rampant political pundits, critics, competitors in businesses, or even strangers on the internet, pointing fingers. And by guilty, I mean, you are hurting your self, your own spirit, your own mind and thought patterns. Being negative, critical, and judgmental is going against the Laws of the Universe. Judging a person does not define who they are; it defines who you are. Continually focusing on the negative turns you negative and reinforces the paradigm within *your mind*. That paradigm, your present conditioning, controls the results in your life. How? Glad you asked.

"A paradigm is a multitude of habits that are fixed in your mind."

~ Bob Proctor

Yes, HABITS. Your paradigm is the mental programing, the operational system, that has nearly absolute control over your habitual behavior. P.S. Most of our behavior is habitual! And most of those habits came from our environment, accumulated and inherited from other people's habits, opinions, and belief systems.

Criticism, judging, or the fear of being criticized or judged is nothing more than an *ignorant habit*, picked up and developed somewhere along life's way. Even as I first wrote the words in this chapter, I had to squash the fear that tried to raise its ugly head within me; the fear of criticism and judgment, the fear that I may come off as too harsh in this chapter. I told that fear-thought to take a hike. I have spent decades developing my self-worth, courage, and awareness; that measly little weasel of a thought was easy to recognize, and even easier to expel because I frequently exercise my choice to be courageous. Like a pop-up-whacka-game at a child's carnival; I keenly watch for negative thoughts that may pop up, then I quickly bang them away with my mental courage mallet. This may sound silly to you, but the visual makes me laugh, and it works!

To live in a glass house is often used as a figure of speech referring to *vulnerability*. "Living in a glass house" can represent one's impression of living in transparency, open to judgment, and criticism. There are no closets to hide in, when you live in a glass house. Which brings me to a story, shared with permission by my dear friend, Kevin Smith. He knows a thing or two about glass houses *and* closets.

Kevin, like myself, was raised in a lower middle-class family, framed in the black and white world of the late 1950s and '60s. Neither of us suffered poverty; there just weren't a lot of "extras" when we were growing up. We were each blessed with loving parents who provided food, clothing, and shelter on a tight budget, along with a stable family life, and were supported in a fishbowl of family and like-minded friends. In fact, Kevin and I were both experienced having been raised in the same rigid denomination of religion. We grew up being taught that if you deviated in the slightest bit from the "straight and narrow path" of this doctrine, then you were going to hell. Do not pass GO, do not collect $200. We were also taught not just to respect authority, but to *fear* authority, to fear God. Fear was a core value in our religion and in our family creed. Fear of God, fear of authority, and fear of what the neighbors might think.

One of many things than Kevin and I share in common from our childhoods is our imagination during play time. Back in a simpler era before all of the electronic diversions of today, we kids had to rely on our imagination to entertain ourselves. One of my favorite pastimes was playing with dolls. I especially loved Barbie. So did Kevin.

Kevin "played dolls", as we used to refer to it, along with his younger sister. His G.I. Joe doll was invited to the party. I can recall "borrowing" my younger brother's action figure doll for imaginary escapades with my dolls. They all had bendable knees and could ride in his Jeep! Okay, so I borrowed the Jeep, too. I built them an imaginary house, using a small box with doorways cut out of the cardboard walls. It had adjacent rooms whose walls were made of books, tissue boxes, or anything else my imagination visualized for their dwelling. It turned out differently every time I built it, but that was half the fun! There was never a ceiling.

There *was* a ceiling, however, in Kevin's doll world. Although his mom encouraged doll-play for both of her children's development and his dad never said anything, Kevin began to pick up on a sense that there was something wrong with little boys playing with dolls. It could have been the social norm of the time, or the strictness of our religion, but little Kevin began to hide his love of dolls and other "girl's stuff" as he grew older. He began living a double life, of sorts, downplaying his interests and pretending to follow the polarizing opinions of others. I understand. I, too, was raised with a certain code of conduct that dictated which toys were for boys, and which ones were for girls. I didn't like those rules. I played with cars, cap-guns, and made roadways in our gravel driveway with my brother's construction trucks. I loved cars! I collected small, dye-cast models, and loved it when Daddy would sometimes "go fast" on a backroad (now I drive my own fast car). I perceived the same sort of, "there's something not quite right" vibe from my parents for loving cars, being a grease monkey and a tomboy, as Kevin felt for his hours of role-playing with dolls and friends.

In 1927, *Time* magazine printed a chart showing sex-appropriate colors for girls and boys, according to leading U.S. stores. In the 1940s, manufacturers settled on pink for girls and blue for boys, so Baby Boomers like Kevin and myself were raised with that binary which was foisted onto children by society and church. Males and females were expected to play certain roles. And, not just with toys or clothing, but with a gender bias on behavior, expectations, and career assumptions. I love that Kevin and I blurred the lines of those social and religious paradigms.

Around age 40, I had a spiritual enlightenment. I have been studying ever since that awakening. Oddly, Kevin had an epiphany at age 40 as well. In both cases, we each had to summon our courage to ultimately make choices that were fearful and consequential.

As children, we all grow older, mature a bit, and discover our sexuality by the time we are in our teens. Kevin discovered that although he did date females and enjoyed their company, he was more attracted to males. He kept this inside, fearing retribution from the church, disappointment from his family, and ridicule from his classmates. It was clearly made unacceptable by all social and religious pronouncements of the times. He thought, "Well, maybe this is something I will get over". Aaaaaand, it wasn't.

By the time he graduated college, Kevin had secretly dated a few young men. He disguised his true nature from his friends and acquaintances by pretending to have girlfriends or eluding to "dating someone" without mentioning gender. His naturally friendly, adventurous, outgoing personality put him in a lot of social circles on campus, all of whom were unaware of his personal preference.

Hired in the mid-'80s, Kevin found his career in California with an incredible job at an amazing company. Homosexuality was definitely frowned upon, and the label could certainly jeopardize one's job, even in the more progressive city of Los Angeles. As the years went by, he began moving up the ranks. With each promotion or stock option, his anxiety grew, silently. Kevin kept his truth to himself, developing a double life without any real awareness of what that does to one's psyche.

In California, where you live and where you work can be miles and hours apart. Kevin had one life with his career, business related friends, contacts, and after hour social gatherings, and an entirely separate, secondary life that was centered around his sexuality. There was a lot to balance, and a lot to keep track of. He constantly had to check himself, making sure he got his story straight (no pun intended); whom he was sharing information with, whom he was seen with, whom he was hiding from. There was always an undercurrent of fear in his mind; the fear of being "outed", discovered at a gay event, or worse, being captured on film by a television crew. One of Kevin's former colleagues actually *was* captured on TV at a gay rights event; Kevin heard everyone jeer, gossip, and sneer behind his back. The man was completely ostracized. And these were grown-adult professionals, in the 1990s!

In the year 2000, Kevin turned 40. He was in his first, serious, long-term relationship. His career was very profitable.

He was making out financial and personal goal lists and visualizing the beautiful house on a hill that he wanted and the investment returns he was targeting. Due to some changes within the company and the advice of a financial counselor, Kevin had that house within a year and his company offered him a new, lucrative, executive position! He left the security and secrecy of his small, two-bedroom house in L.A., and with bolstered courage, he accepted the offer and he and his partner moved to the Southwestern area of the United States.

You may not be aware of this, but many parts of the Southwestern area have seen prominent advances in lesbian, gay, bisexual, and transgender (LGBT) rights, with homosexuality being legal since the 1970's. Kevin and his partner moved together and found a warmer climate and friendlier atmosphere. Within a year, they had built that beautiful dream house that Kevin had envisioned, a glass house. Set on the top of a hill, the 360-degree views were stunning. It was an incredible, architectural masterpiece, and a testament to visualization and goal setting.

Kevin had his executive title on the line, so he continued his guise as a straight man. The double life he had created was almost second nature by now. After years of life together, Kevin's partner now felt safe enough around Kevin to open up and trust him with his innermost thoughts. Kevin and his partner went to see a therapist one day. The therapist stated to Kevin, "So now let's talk about *you*".

"*Me?* I'm perfect!" Kevin joked. He had gotten very comfortable living this double life; it was all compartmentalized, a little hairy at times to keep it all straight, but nonetheless, he thought he had it all under control. After being prompted by the therapist, though, Kevin bravely opened up about himself and began working with him.

Since Kevin wasn't "out" to anybody but a few, close friends, his partner was feeling "hidden" from everyone. Kevin played the straight game to his friends, his company environment, and his entire family, never once realizing that the glass house he lived in was built by two people. He had become so busy protecting his own life that, despite the fact that he cared very much for his partner, he had somehow missed meeting his needs and cravings to be significant and validated. The pain in both of them was as transparent as the windows on their glass home.

The couple lived in their glass house for several years, each of them working with the therapist at their own, individual pace. Kevin found that this was the impetus, as he did work with his therapist, and started to come out to his world. It was very hard. The fears now barricaded every step of intended growth.

I understand. I've been there. After giving it all that you think you have, having the courage to be authentic has to come from a Higher Source…and, it does show up. You just can't give up before it does. Repeat this pushing of yourself and the "little extra from above", and it builds your wisdom and your faith.

When my husband and I both hit 40 years old (we're only two months apart in age), we both felt a calling, if you will. There was a dissatisfaction in the lack of spirituality in our lives, and a curiosity and hungering that made us think, "There has got to be more to it than this". We began studying religions and philosophy; each of us took our own path but were side by side in the journey. After five years of continual research and study, we decided to change our religious affiliation. We both knew this would not bode well with our families and friends. We converted to Judaism and became closet Jews.

There is a lot of fear that comes with big changes like these. Kevin and I share the experience of that fear. When you make a decision to change, there is instant fear that your relationships will change. You know how your relationships work presently, but it's going to change… on every relationship level. Someone is going to get hurt, someone is going to judge you, condemn you based on their paradigms, and you can't control that. Bodies are going to hit the floor.

For my husband and myself, well, we "laid low" for as long as possible. We both knew the pain, anger, and criticism that would come with our decision. Before we ever converted, I drove over three hours to my parents' home to unburden myself with the news that we had left the church that we'd been raised in. My stomach churned as I rang the doorbell. I was somewhat relieved that only my mother was home for the bombshell. My dad would have blown his cork. I knew this wasn't going to go well. We sat at the kitchen table as I matter-of-factly explained our journey. She didn't condone or understand and began wringing her hands with worry. Unfortunately, that day was the beginning of a 20+ year rift between us.

Studying Judaism was eye-opening. It helped set us free of judging others based on their religious beliefs, or anything for that matter. It set us on a path of spiritual learning and personal growth. It was liberating. Ironically, 20 years later I am way more spiritual than I am religious. I accept people wherever they are, with whatever concept they believe about God. We are all One. We are all connected.

Eventually, when our daughter was getting married by a Rabbi, the folks began to figure things out. We were condemned to hell and declared dead in the church (behind our backs, of course). We lost our large circle of church-going friends and were ostracized by our families. Everyone is a critic. No one wanted to actually sit down and study with us, and we couldn't condense our knowledge into an elevator speech and explain five years of research during a seven-floor ride to the top. That's like asking Albert Einstein, in the car next to you, to explain quantum physics while you're stopped at a traffic light.

Kevin experienced a tremendous fear of telling his parents that he was gay. Gratefully, he attributes his healing to the work he did with his therapist who helped him to become more authentic. The entire body of therapy work was done under the banner of being authentic to his world. This sound advice plays out in so many ways; it's not just about being gay, or about a certain religion; this is about everything, *whoever you are.* Yes, coming out as a gay man or lesbian woman is an exaggerated example of being more authentic, but this lesson really applies to so many more people and situations.

So, here's Kevin, living in his glass mansion, with no closet to hide in anymore. His partner and his therapist encouraged him to tell his parents the truth, that he'd been living a lie; not for their sake, but for his own righteousness. He went home to his parents for a four-day weekend. He spent those four days playing mind games with himself, coming up with reasons and excuses for why he couldn't tell them. On the last evening of his visit, he realized he was out of time. He mustered every ounce of courage he could and went into the living room where his folks sat. Taking in a deep breath, he began.

"Guys, I need to tell you what's going on here". They were a bit alarmed. "What? What?" they inquired, with concern. It was now or never. With that extra bit of courage from our Higher Source, Kevin gushed, "I have a partner, and I'm gay". Kevin's parents showered him with love. They both exclaimed,

"Well, that explains it!", as they rose to embrace him. His mom cried for him, hurt for realizing he had to keep this inside of himself for 41 years. For Kevin, this was a liberating, beautiful experience. He had been so worried about his dad's reaction, that his news would disappoint his dad, or that somehow his being gay would be a poor reflection of his dad's fathering skills or challenge his manhood. Interestingly, his dad took the news better than his mom!

Kevin had been so concerned about his parents' feelings, but love prevailed. Their love for him prevailed over everything. There was no judgment, no condemnation, no "let's try and fix this" attitude. They accepted him; "This is who you are". Some of our family and friends eventually came to understand that our conversion to Judaism didn't change "who we are". It expanded us, opened our minds, opened our understanding. They returned to be a part of our lives once again, for which my husband and I are both grateful.

When you are your authentic self and people have a problem with that, then that is *their* problem, not yours. As Bob Proctor teaches, "Being offended is a choice". Ask yourself, what is it that you want to get, ultimately, from taking that courageous step forward? For Kevin, it truly was about being his more authentic self. For all of us, we *must* have the courage to say, like Kevin, "You know what? Being on *this* side of it all is *far* better than being on the previous side, where I was in pain and denial, living a lie. It is so much better living to be authentic and living in Truth".

It takes courage to get you from point A to point B. Build your courage through seeing the benefit, the outcome. Building courage through desire for something different; the longing and hungering that moves a person to take action and make a change. Our old paradigms will try and push us down and suppress that bubbling spring of courage with negative thoughts like, "No, no, no, let me protect you. You don't need to do this". That little child who lives in our subconscious mind can often be scared, fearful, and hurt. As Kevin's therapist taught him, it's time for adult Kevin to have a conversation with little Kevin.

"Calmness of mind is one of the beautiful jewels of wisdom. It is the result of long and patient effort in self-control."

~ James Allen

The next time you experience anxiety or fear, get in a quiet place, close your eyes, and picture your youngest self. Calm yourself. Control your thoughts. Breathe in peace and courage, and calmly tell your little child within that you've got this. Any time fear tries to raise its ugly head, you repeat to your inner child, "You know what? I've got this", over and over. You will be amazed at the power of your subconscious mind.

I am proud of my brother-from-another-mother, Kevin. I am happy that he chose to move out of the glass house he was living in, and into a more authentic life, filled with love acceptance, and faith. We each grew up in our experiences to become who we are supposed to be today. Namaste.

TEN

A Letter About Moral Courage

Moral courage is defined as the ability to act rightly in the face of popular opposition. It is a commitment to moral principles, with an awareness of a vulnerability, or the possible dangers involved with supporting those principles, and a willingness to risk that danger. Moral courage is driven by principle and involves deliberation and, often, careful thought.

My Dearest Readers,

For many of us, when we were young, our developing moral courage may have been primed by instances of peer pressure of doing something against our "knowing better". The allure of sneaking a smoke or under-age drinking, stealing something on a dare, or even experimenting with drugs, provoked a conscious choice to give in or muster the courage to say no. Perhaps our moral courage grew as we resisted cheating on a test in school or made a choice to walk away from a fight, not to lie to our mamma or steal change from Nana's coin purse. For some of us, the fear of the consequences of being caught, the humiliation, or punishments of such juvenile transgressions was enough to keep us in line. *Sometimes exercising restraint requires more courage than taking action.* Nevertheless, our young, moral courage, however employed, was the beginning of building our self-respect and a foundation for our personal integrity, before we even fully understood the definition. Our emotions and feelings should tell us enough… when we do the right thing, it feels good.

More and more these days, courage is showing up in young people in the form of those who stand up to bullies, defend the weak, and are charitable with their understanding and caring of others. Moral courage is not driven by fear, but by a sense of right, a sense of respect for others and themselves, and an internal universal code of Right. These young people aren't heroes in the sense of military personnel, law enforcement or other first responders; however, there are plenty of instances of incredible acts of heroism, bravery, and compassion; inspirational and courageous deeds, *because it was the right thing to do.*

When we mature as adults, our moral courage is further defined in our personal relationships, in the integrity of our business dealings, and even in our political views. It is demonstrated in our actions, our words, and how we conduct our lives. We live by our personal code of ethics, which began its formation when we were children, and literally continues to either develop or dwindle, right up to today. Our internal code of conduct is apparent in how we show up in our commitments, our passions, our business models, our families, and our spiritual growth and understanding. It is answering the call to do the Right thing, with a clear comprehension of sticking to our principles, and damn the torpedoes. When we stay open and receptive, when we are aware that we continuously create our environment with our thoughts, attitude, and emotions, then we are in vast favor of constant improvement and personal growth.

"Lack of courage is lack of knowledge."

~ Rachel Bazzy

Lack of courage is being anxious, fearful, faint-hearted, nervous, panicky, weak, timid, afraid, and spiritless. Lack of courage means an insufficiency, a shortage, or an absence of courage that is desired or required. Lack of courage is lack of knowledge; the knowledge of the Laws of the Universe, and how to use them. *Ignorance* is not bliss; it is cowardice.

I will go deeper. Suicide is not courageous. Suicide or attempted suicide is a form of mental ignorance. It is dis-ease in the mind. Please allow me to explain what I mean.

Psychology Today decrees that there are six reasons why people attempt suicide. Some people are psychotic, listening to the inner voices that often command them to self-destruct. Others are impulsive, their attempts often related to drugs and alcohol. Some are crying out for help; they don't know how to get it any other way. There are a few who have a philosophical desire to die, based on a reasoned decision often motivated by a painful, terminal illness. They want to take control of their destiny, alleviating their suffering. And then there are those who have made a mistake, either through an accidental, lethal ingestion of something or perhaps from experimenting with oxygen deprivation.

Accordingly, the number one reason that people attempt suicide is that they are depressed. Bob Proctor explains how a person arrives at the low level of thinking, called depression, in the following lesson. I will paraphrase.

We have two choices, IGNORANCE or KNOWLEDGE.

When someone is *ignorant* and has no understanding, no awareness, they live in a state of worry and doubt. Worry and doubt soon turn into fear. Fear grows into anxiety. Anxiety is suppressed, which turns into depression. Depression, unchecked and fed with self-pity, guilt, low esteem thoughts, cowardice and ungratefulness, turns into *disease*. The person is not at ease; they have a *dis-ease*. From there it goes to disintegration and, you guessed it, suicide.

> *"Faith is the ability to see the invisible – to believe in the incredible. That is what enables you to receive what the masses think is impossible."*
>
> ~ Clarence Smithson

Stick with me, now, because this gets better on the other side of the thinking. KNOWLEDGE comes from studying and understanding. This builds our faith; our faith in the Laws of the Universe and faith in ourselves. Faith leads to a sense of well-being. There is an *expression* of this well-being, which leads to a further acceleration. We are then at ease and live in a state of creation.

Nothing is impossible to the mind. Our thoughts cause everything. Having the courage to explore these thoughts and teachings will help you to realize that you can take control of your own life, beginning today, with a commitment to growth. If you have a thought, right now, that says this is bull muffins, then say hello to your little friend, the paradigm. That sucker will lie to you, in an attempt to "protect" you. Don't let it win. Don't listen to the dark conversation, the negative thoughts that rob you of your happiness.

It is my honor to share these stories and lessons of courage with you. My goal is to give you something to think about, something to contemplate, something to examine your heart about. Courage is the most important virtue we need to develop within ourselves. Master courage, and anything is possible.

With Love and Courage,

Rachel

ABOUT THE AUTHOR

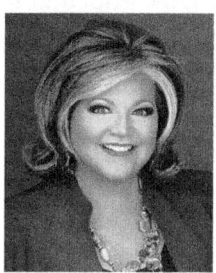

Photograph: Tommy Collier

Rachel Bazzy, an extremely creative being who has dedicated her life to being of service, has influenced countless lives with her thoughtful writings, empathic strength, and developed courage. As a businesswoman for over 30 years, she has an established reputation for integrity, valor, and honesty. She is energetic in the studies of personal growth, emotional, spiritual, and psychological development, and passionate about empowering others to realize and develop the virtue of courage in their own lives.

To learn more, visit www.rachelbazzy.com

The **Unstoppable Foundation** is a
non-profit humanitarian organization
bringing sustainable education to children and
communities in developing countries thereby
creating a safer and more just world for everyone.

Our Mission:
To ensure EVERY child has access to the
life-long gift of an education.

It's not charity, it's empowerment.

Learn more at UnstoppableFoundation.org

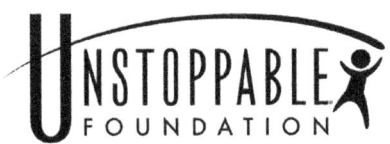

For more information
about Rachel Bazzy and *Courage*

Website
www.rachelbazzy.com

Facebook
Rachel Bazzy, Master of Courage

Email
rachel@rachelbazzy.com

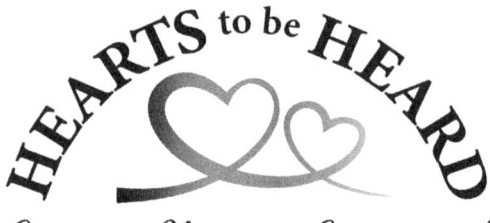

Giving a Voice to Creativity!

Your donation will give a voice to the creativity
that lies within the hearts of physically,
spiritually and mentally challenged children.

By helping us publish their books,
musical creations and works of art you will
make a difference in a child's life;
a child who would not otherwise be heard.

Donate now by going to

HeartstobeHeard.com

The children thank you!!

Made in the USA
Coppell, TX
16 April 2020